To Improve Health and Health Care

Volume XI

Stephen L. Isaacs and

David C. Colby, Editors

Foreword by Risa Lavizzo-Mourey

To Improve Health and Health Care

Volume XI

The Robert Wood Johnson Foundation Anthology

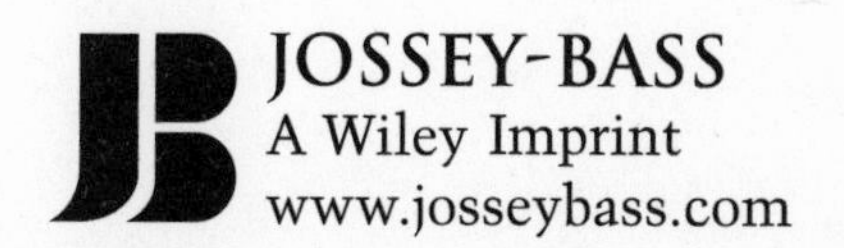

Published by Jossey-Bass
A Wiley Imprint
989 Market Street, San Francisco, CA 94103-1741—www.josseybass.com

Jossey-Bass books and products are available through most bookstores. To contact Jossey-Bass directly call our Customer Care Department within the U.S. at 800-956-7739, outside the U.S. at 317-572-3986, or fax 317-572-4002.

Jossey-Bass also publishes its books in a variety of electronic formats. Some content that appears in print may not be available in electronic books.

Cataloging-in-Publication data on file with the Library of Congress.

ISBN 978-0-7879-8638-4

Printed in the United States of America
FIRST EDITION
PB Printing 10 9 8 7 6 5 4 3 2 1

Table of Contents

Tables of Contents of Previous Volumes

Foreword

Risa Lavizzo-Mourey

In his comprehensive examination of the nation's foundations, Joel Fleishman, the former president of the Atlantic Philanthropic Service Company—the U.S. affiliate of the Atlantic Philanthropies—praised the contributions of foundations in benefiting the public and improving society, but warned that "what they have not done is to create a climate of transparency, the lack of which both causes foundations to underperform their potential and creates growing public distrust."[1] To stem this underperformance and suspicion, Fleishman urges foundations to "introduce a greater degree of transparency and accountability into [their] world."

As a matter of principle, the board and leadership of the Robert Wood Johnson Foundation have always taken the position that the organization should be hardheaded in evaluating the results of its programs and generous in sharing its findings with the public.[2] Even though the Robert Wood Johnson Foundation is a private philanthropy, we consider it to be a public trust, with a responsibility to be as accountable for our programs as we are for our finances.

Over the years, the Foundation has developed a variety of ways to evaluate the impact of its initiatives and to share information about its activities widely. Our grant results reports unit has posted more than two thousand summaries of Foundation-supported programs and projects on our Web site. The Web site itself contains a wealth of information about the Foundation, and it has recently been redesigned to make it easier for visitors to navigate. We ask our grantees to disseminate the results of their work widely, and we encourage our staff to share their knowledge by writing articles and making conference presentations.

Three years ago, in collaboration with Jossey-Bass, a San Francisco-based publishing house, we began a new book series to give readers a better understanding of the best work done in fields that the foundation has nurtured—such as school health, generalist medicine, and tobacco control policy.[3] That policy series complements this *To Improve Health and Health Care: The Robert Wood Johnson Foundation Anthology* series, also published by Jossey-Bass.

Now in its eleventh year, the *Anthology* series is a unique vehicle through which the Foundation shares information with the public and with the fields in which we work; distributing twelve thousand copies to leaders and practitioners in the health, policy, and philanthropy communities. In each volume, outside evaluators and outstanding writers offer unbiased assessments of fields and programs in which the Foundation has invested, and, in some cases, members of our staff present the inside story of why and how the Foundation chose certain paths to address health issues and policies. We hope that readers will learn from the *Anthology* what the Foundation and its grantees did, why they did it, and what they learned from the experience. In some cases, our work will be deemed successful; in others, the results will be less positive. Whatever the outcomes, a frank, unalloyed examination will lead to greater understanding and lessons that can be applied in the future.

Although I generally do not single out specific chapters, I found several in this year's volume of particular interest. These include Carolyn Newbergh's chapter on the Foundation's efforts to promote high-quality health care in an environment that offers few incentives to provide such care; Paul Jellinek's chapter on our work to develop programs of sufficient scale to improve the health and safety of a significant number of urban children at a time when government had reduced its role; Susan McGrath's chapter on our Active Living programs that encourage walking and biking through better urban planning; and Jim Knickman and Kelly Hunt's chapter on our efforts to evaluate the impact of our philanthropic investments.

Fleishman writes that "the various sins committed by foundations—arrogance, discourtesy, inaccessibility, and the others—result from their lack of accountability." We trust that readers of this *Anthology* will note that we take seriously our responsibility to be open and transparent about measuring and reporting on the impact of the work we are privileged to be able to undertake.

Risa Lavizzo-Mourey
President and CEO
The Robert Wood Johnson Foundation
Princeton, New Jersey
October 2007

Notes

1. Fleishman, J. L. *The Foundation: A Great American Secret.* New York: Public Affairs Press, 2007.
2. Fleishman singled out the Robert Wood Johnson Foundation, along with the Wallace and Packard foundations, as philanthropies that have been at the forefront of transparency and accountability.
3. Isaacs, S. L., and Knickman, J. R. *Generalist Medicine and the U.S. Health System.* San Francisco: Jossey-Bass, 2004; Graham Lear, J., Isaacs, S. L., and Knickman, J. R. *School Health Services and Programs.* San Francisco: Jossey-Bass, 2006; and Warner, K. E. *Tobacco Control Policy.* San Francisco: Jossey-Bass, 2006.

Editors' Introduction

Stephen L. Isaacs and David C. Colby

This year's volume of *The Robert Wood Johnson Foundation Anthology* illustrates several approaches that the Foundation employs to improve health and health care in the United States and to measure its impact.

Seeding and nurturing new fields is one approach that has characterized the Foundation's grantmaking since its very beginning in 1972. Previous volumes have explored the Foundation's efforts to build the fields of nursing and nurse practitioners, tobacco control, and end-of-life care.[1] This year's *Anthology* contains two chapters related to field building.

We lead off Volume XI with a chapter by journalist Carolyn Newbergh that examines the Foundation's work to improve quality of care. Though quality has been a priority of the Foundation through most of its history, its contribution to building this field has not been widely recognized. This chapter weaves the various strands of the Foundation's many quality-improvement programs into a comprehensive tapestry. In Chapter Two, David Colby, the Foundation's vice president for research and evaluation (and the coeditor of this volume), tells the story of how the Foundation helped create and develop the field of health services research. Colby traces the Foundation's efforts—from subsidizing the research of a few "great men" to developing and honing fellowship programs and, ultimately, supporting a few key institutions and the journal *Health Affairs*.

The next three chapters focus on the Foundation's work to address important health challenges. In Chapter Three, Will Bunch, a journalist, looks at the Foundation's programs to reduce teenage pregnancy. Particularly revealing is Bunch's exploration of how the Foundation has tackled such a volatile and divisive social issue over the years. Smoking by pregnant women—many of whom are young and poor—carries serious health risks for both the fetus and the woman herself. In Chapter Four, Fen Montaigne, a freelance writer, delves into Smoke-Free Families, a program that funded research to understand how to help pregnant women stop smoking and then to introduce successful smoking-cessation methods into routine prenatal care. Chapter Five examines the way that one community is addressing a serious gap in the health care system—the fact that people with mental illnesses who are also substance abusers are treated by separate components of the health care system. This chapter, written by journalist Paul Brodeur, describes an experimental project in Fort Collins, Colorado, that is trying to coordinate the treatment of individuals who are both mentally ill and addicted to drugs or alcohol.

Good or poor health is, for the most part, caused by nonhealth factors, including behavior, lifestyle choices, the social and economic environment (for example, education, race, social class, income, ethnicity, neighborhood), and genes. The next three chapters examine a series of initiatives to improve health by addressing its determinants. What characterizes these programs is their broad, indirect approaches to improving health—approaches that go beyond ones usually considered within the purview of health philanthropy.

The Foundation's portfolio of Active Living grants, discussed by freelance journalist Susan McGrath in Chapter Six, has attempted to encourage people to get more physical activity by making the "built environment" more friendly to walking and bicycling. In doing so, the Foundation and its grantees collaborated with urban planners, architects, school crossing guards, zoning boards, environmentalists, and others outside of the Foundation's usual partners.

In the Urban Health Initiative, described by former Foundation vice president Paul Jellinek in Chapter Seven, the Foundation attempted to improve the well-being of children by funding such activities as afterschool educational and athletic programs, park and playground improvement, and adult mentoring. The focus on improving the life chances of disadvantaged children—as contrasted with a focus directly on their health—went beyond traditional approaches to health improvement and, like the Active Living programs, led to collaborations with government officials, school administrators and teachers, budget analysts, city planners, transportation experts, and others who were typically outside the normal orbit of health agencies and health philanthropy.

The conceptual grounds for this holistic approach toward children's well-being comes from something called *positive youth development.* This theory—that a caring adult can strengthen the natural resiliency of children living in difficult circumstances, afford them stability, serve as a role models, and provide guidance through hard times—underpins a variety of Foundation-funded mentoring programs. In Chapter Eight, Irene Wielawski, a freelance journalist, examines these programs, which range from after-school sports projects in the San Francisco Bay Area and Boston to long-term, one-on-one mentoring by adults who receive a salary equivalent to that of a schoolteacher.

The last two chapters get inside the world of philanthropy. In Chapter Nine, James Knickman, former vice president for research and evaluation at the Foundation, and Kelly Hunt, a former Foundation research officer, describe the ways that the Robert Wood Johnson Foundation evaluates its own programs and their impact. This is one of those chapters that attempts to demystify philanthropy by describing the internal processes and thinking of the Foundation. It is especially germane at a time when foundations throughout the United States have become increasingly motivated to measure and clarify their effectiveness to audiences outside their world. The final chapter, by the author Digby Diehl, explores how the Robert Wood Johnson Foundation played a leadership role in the development of sports philanthropy. Through the Sports Philanthropy Project, the Robert Wood Johnson Foundation was able to offer expertise in effective grantmaking to foundations and other charities established and supported by professional sports teams.

The chapters in this year's volume reveal much about both approaches to improving health and health care and the ways that one foundation operates. Taken as a whole, we hope that the book continues to fulfill what Risa Lavizzo-Mourey termed in her foreword as the Foundation's "responsibility to be as accountable for our programs as it is for our finances."

Stephen L. Isaacs, San Francisco, California
David C. Colby, Princeton, New Jersey
October 2007

Notes

1. Isaacs, S. L., and Knickman, J. R. *Generalist Medicine and the U.S. Health System.* San Francisco: Jossey-Bass, 2004; Graham Lear, J., Isaacs, S. L., and Knickman, J. R. *School Health Services and Programs.* San Francisco: Jossey-Bass, 2006; and Warner, K. E. *Tobacco Control Policy.* San Francisco: Jossey-Bass, 2006.

Acknowledgments

We would like to begin by expressing our appreciation to Pat Crow, whose mastery of his craft demonstrates why he is widely considered to be a legendary editor. His contributions to this and to all previous volumes of the *Anthology* have been enormous.

We owe a debt of gratitude to many more people. Outside of the Robert Wood Johnson Foundation, the external review committee—Susan Dentzer, Bill Morrill, Patti Patrizi, and Jon Showstack—again provided us with great wisdom in their review of chapter drafts. Carolyn Shea proved herself to be an extraordinary fact checker. Ty Baldwin and Lauren MacIntryre were highly professional in entering editorial changes and presenting us with clean manuscripts. We extend our gratitude to Andy Pasternack, Seth Schwartz, Kelsey McGee, and others at Jossey-Bass who shepherded the book through print production.

Within the Robert Wood Johnson Foundation, special thanks are due to David Morse, who plays a role akin to a third coeditor although he is not publicly credited for it, and to Risa Lavizzo-Mourey, whose respect for the integrity of the *Anthology* makes it possible for it to be open and unbiased. Molly McKaughan did her usual splendid job of critiquing every chapter, aided this year on one chapter by her colleague in the grant results reporting unit, Marian Bass. Edie Burbank-Schmitt provided invaluable research assistance, and Hinda Feige Greenberg, Mary Beth Kren, and Barbara Sergeant were most efficient in finding books and articles that the authors and we needed. Deb Malloy, Sherry DeMarchi, Tina Hines, and Chris Clayton made coordination between the San Francisco-based editor and the staff members at the Foundation seem easy. Marilyn Ernst was extremely conscientious in handling administrative matters, as were Mary Castria, Ellen Coyote, Carol Owle, Carolyn Sholer, and Chris Sowa in handling financial matters. Hope Woodhead and Barbara Sherwood oversaw production and distribution with their usual aplomb.

We also owe a debt of gratitude to those people who were gracious enough to review drafts of individual chapters: Nancy Barrand, Terry Bazzarre, Adam Coyne, Nancy Fishman, Sue Hassmiller, Jane Lowe, Jim Knickman, Kate Kraft, Jim Marks, Joe Marx, Tracy Orleans, Steve Schroeder, Polly Seitz, Judy Stavisky, and Anne Weiss.

Finally, special thanks are due to Elizabeth Dawson, research and editorial director at Health Policy Associates, who plays a critical role in the entire *Anthology* process—handling everything from reviewing manuscripts and serving as liaison between authors and editors to supervising the production process and taking care of the administrative and financial matters.

S.L.I. and D.C.C.

CHAPTER 1

Improving Quality of Care

Carolyn Newbergh

Editors' Introduction

Over the past fifteen years, Americans have become aware that they are not receiving medical care of the highest quality. Concern about quality surfaced in the 1990s with suspicions that managed care companies were skimping on care to increase the bottom line. It resurfaced, in a different way, in the early 2000s with the publication of a widely reported Institute of Medicine study finding that faulty care in hospitals was responsible for between 44,000 and 98,000 avoidable deaths a year[1] and a well-publicized report by Elizabeth McGlynn and her colleagues indicating that more than half of chronically ill patients do not receive appropriate care.[2]

The movement to improve the quality of healthcare is a response to these kinds of concerns, and the Robert Wood Johnson Foundation, which has been concerned about quality since the 1970s, has helped to create and establish the movement. The Foundation did not advertise its work to improve quality of care, and until recently it was not a priority area. Perhaps because quality-of-care grantmaking was carried out within the context of chronic care (which *was* a priority), many staff members did not even recognize that the Foundation was doing so much to improve quality. In this chapter, Carolyn Newbergh, a freelance journalist and frequent contributor to the *Anthology* series, chronicles the Foundation's efforts to improve the quality of medical care in the United States.

This chapter can be read in two ways. One of them is through a public health lens: the recognition that the quality of medical care in the United States is not all that it is cracked up to be and the efforts to change that. The other is through a philanthropy lens. Quality is an area, like health services research, tobacco control, and end-of-life care, where the Foundation has spurred the creation of a field. It did so by funding research, strengthening the capacity of researchers, financing demonstration projects, developing standards, supporting professional organizations, and backing champions who have played and continue to play critical leadership roles.

Notes

1. Institute of Medicine. *To Err Is Human: Building a Safer Health System.* Washington, D.C.: National Academies Press, 2000.
2. McGlynn, E., and others. "The Quality of Health Care Delivered to Adults in the United States." *New England Journal of Medicine,* 2003, *348*(26), 2635–2645.

Rebecca Bryson knew that she was a complicated patient, but still, she thought that the health care system in Whatcom County, Washington, should be able to do better for her than it did. She had congestive heart failure, diabetes, anemia, gastrointestinal bleeding, and various serious complications, was being treated by fourteen doctors, and was taking forty-two medications. During her hospitalizations, she was repeatedly given the wrong drug because her various specialists weren't kept abreast of the latest changes others had made. At times, she received medications that she was allergic to or that were intended for someone else. When she was out of the hospital, she had the hardest time getting through to tell her doctor about worrisome symptoms—she had to present a compelling enough case to the receptionist for her to pass her consultation request on to the nurse. Then she had to make a convincing case to the nurse—and once more, if lucky, repeat it all to the doctor. Adding insult to injury, each time she was hospitalized she was served meat. She's a vegetarian.

"Being sick is hard work," she told a rapt audience during a health care conference.

Bryson's complaints fell on receptive ears. Led by a doctor and a nurse with a passion for improving health care quality, a community coalition of health care organizations in Whatcom County took Bryson's struggles and those of many other patients and families to heart and turned them into a plan as part of the Robert Wood Johnson Foundation's Pursuing Perfection grant initiative. Pursuing Perfection was designed to attack just this kind of system malfunction and breakdown.

The Whatcom County team took as its main goal putting patients—particularly those with chronic illnesses—at the center of the communitywide health care system. Patients and family members took seats on committees to redesign health care processes, and their ideas were treated as gems to be mined. They helped develop two big innovations: the "shared care plan" and the "clinical care specialist." The shared care plan was a way to manage the care of patients with chronic illnesses; it contained the patient's diagnoses, medications, lab work results, allergies, lifestyle goals, names of providers, and advance directives. Unlike the normal physician-ordered plan, however, this one was devised in collaboration with and controlled by the patient. Since it was available both online to all providers within the Whatcom community system and on paper, patients could tote their plan with them anywhere.

"It really appeals to people that you can travel someplace like Seattle or Pittsburgh or Bangladesh and have all your medical information available," said Conrad Grabow, one of many patients who, with his wife, contributed suggestions for improving hospital processes from the patient's perspective.

The clinical care specialist—or "coach/navigator"—ran interference for the patient, breaking down barriers put up by gatekeepers in the physicians' offices. With access to doctors' own inner phone lines and offices, these nurses or social workers would get vital information that patients needed quickly so their condition wouldn't deteriorate or land them in the emergency department. The coach/navigator also educated the patients, helping them to make lifestyle changes and to minimize setbacks at various stages of their illness.

The program reduced both hospitalizations and medication errors—and resulted in an average cost saving of $3,000 on each of the sixty-nine patients who participated. "What we learned, I think, is transformative," said Marc Pierson, the physician who oversaw the Whatcom County grant. "We learned that patients and their small social networks giving support are incredibly ready to help with their health. Health care policy in America is completely devoid of the concept of a patient, a real human being who makes choices and has behavior change. They're viewed as just cost and liability. They're as invisible as black people were in the thirties, forties, and fifties."

Quality Moves onto the National Agenda

Americans everywhere are subject to the dangerous vagaries of the health care system: uncoordinated care that leaves patients open to too many mistakes, care that falls short of what science tells us is the best treatment, little recognition that the patient's active involvement is invaluable to the healing process, and almost no use of the information technology that has transformed the world outside of health care. Too many people have had mammograms misplaced, the wrong limb operated on, or the wrong dosage of a drug given.

At the dawn of the twenty-first century, however, a nationwide movement to improve health care quality was attracting considerable attention. "In the area of quality, there's probably been more traction gained than in anywhere else in health care over the last ten or fifteen years," said Gail Warden, president emeritus of the Henry Ford Health System in Detroit, who has played numerous important roles during what many are beginning to call a revolution. He is also a former Robert Wood Johnson Foundation trustee.

For much of the previous century, it was simply assumed that American health care was the best in the world and that doctors didn't need anyone meddling in how they approached their practice. Besides, doctors often said medicine was both an art and a science, and quality was not something that could be dictated or defined. In 1910, the Flexner Report directed the profession to base the education of physicians on scientifically proven treatments, and for many decades that seemed to suffice. There were efforts to improve quality—professional standards review organizations, quality assurance committees, and criteria established by the Joint Commission on Accreditation of Hospitals (now the Joint Commission)—but physicians were largely left alone. It was only in the 1990s, with the widespread adoption of managed care and the concern that managed care companies were skimping on care to fatten the bottom line, that the situation began to change.

Although the longtime confidence about American health care persisted, the people at the front lines knew a different story. The doctors and the nurses had what amounted to a closely guarded secret among themselves about the dangers patients faced, especially when it came to hospital care. Although pharmaceutical breakthroughs and technology were leading to longer lives, they were also adding complexity and increasing the ways in which the system could break down. "I think every one of us, every doctor and nurse, we've known since training how unsafe health care is," Marc Pierson said.

One would think such widespread uneasiness would lead to change. Instead, there was a medical culture that simply didn't want to believe it. "Any time a health care professional or patient runs into a bad outcome, one is always predisposed to think it was natural causes, it could not have been avoided, and not that you screwed up," said Arnold Milstein, the medical director of the Pacific Business Group on Health and a cofounder of the Leapfrog Group, a consortium of employers working to improve the quality and reduce the cost of medical care. "That's why this went on so long—there was not a good read on exactly how unreliable the quality of health care was."

Beginning in the 1980s, research—some of it supported by the Robert Wood Johnson Foundation—began documenting the fact that American medical care was not what it should be. Studies by Robert Brook at the RAND Corporation found variations in the way patients were treated depending on where they lived. John Wennberg at Dartmouth Medical School found that patients with the same health conditions received different treatment depending on the region of the country they lived in.[1] In the 1990s, RAND compiled a review of the literature on health care quality that showed substantial underuse, overuse, and misuse of medical services, exposing patients to more harm than good. These research efforts landed with a muffled thud; the public was not paying attention, and the myth of the preeminence of American medical care continued.

In the late 1990s and early 2000s, the disturbing secret about health care quality began to receive national attention with the publication of two landmark reports by the Institute of Medicine (IOM). In 1999, *To Err Is Human: Building a Safer Health System* put out a chilling statistic: up to ninety-eight thousand people die *unnecessarily* each year in American hospitals because of medical errors. These are from incidents in which the wrong dosage of medication is given, infections lead to fatal pneumonias, and—the kind of error that always commands headlines—operations are performed on the wrong person or body part.[2] *To Err Is Human* is universally described as a "wake-up call." The public learned—in real numbers—that this was not just a matter of isolated anecdotes but that danger lurked for *everyone* admitted to a hospital.

"When you put a number on something, it allows people to see that this is more than the number of people who die from breast cancer and auto accidents each year," said Janet Corrigan, who, as the lead staff member of the IOM Committee on Quality of Health Care in America, drafted much of the report; she now heads the National Quality Forum. "We wanted folks to understand the magnitude of the problem."

Two years later, the IOM's second report on quality and safety, *Crossing the Quality Chasm: A New Health System for the 21st Century,* which the Robert Wood Johnson Foundation partially funded, reported that a huge divide exists between the care that patients should receive and the care that they get.[3] Physicians can't keep up with the flood of medical research and are taking up to seventeen years to incorporate new information into their practice. Patient care processes are badly designed and uncoordinated, sorely lacking the information technology that could reduce waste and help in tracking patients' needs. Care for chronic illnesses accounts for nearly 70 percent of health care spending, but services in the community are inadequate to help patients manage their conditions. Furthermore, the payment system rewards providers for doing more, including correcting their own mistakes, rather than for good outcomes. *The Quality Chasm* also introduced to a broad audience the notion that health care needs to take a page from industry and use its engineering improvement methods to aim for top quality, efficiency, and safety.

"The current care systems cannot do the job," the report said. "Trying harder will not work. Changing systems of care will." *The Quality Chasm* then laid out six goals that would become akin to a mantra for the quality improvement movement that these two reports helped inspire. Care should be "safe, effective, patient-centered, timely, efficient, and equitable." Adding to the case for quality was a seminal study by Elizabeth McGlynn and others at RAND Health, funded by the Robert Wood Johnson Foundation, which found that just 55 percent of adults get health care that meets quality standards.[4]

The movement was off and running, powered by many articulate, passionate, and dedicated leaders and fueled by frontline workers, hospitals, and communities fed up with a system that doesn't serve its customers well enough. It brought with it many new concepts—such as transparency and accountability of performance, Six Sigma industrial improvement principles, total quality improvement, rapid cycle change, and pay for performance.

The reformers were up against enormous odds, with resistance to change probably the biggest impediment. Many providers, policymakers, and administrators regarded this big push as nothing more than a fad and certainly not a science. Some of the movement's leaders, especially the charismatic Donald Berwick, were likened to religious zealots. Critics charged that basing care on protocols or evidence-based medicine—treatment derived from scientific evidence of the most effective approach—reduces health care to "cookbook medicine" rather than the art many have long believed it to be.

The IOM reports instigated a seismic push to transform the lumbering giant that is American health care. Quantifying the damage had struck a nerve. The time was right for reform—to imagine new ways of doing things and to try them out. An October 2006 *Newsweek* report discussed "Fixing America's Hospitals." The Institute for Healthcare Improvement's highly publicized 100,000 Lives Campaign enlisted more than three thousand hospitals to voluntarily reduce common, preventable medical errors and estimated that it saved 122,300 lives over eighteen months.

"There has been a concerted effort by a number of national leaders to raise the quality issues," said RAND's McGlynn. "I do think a growing number of people both recognize that there's a problem and believe that we must do something about it and that we can do something. If that's the essence of a movement, then, yes, that's what it is."

Quality at the Robert Wood Johnson Foundation: Moving from Second to First Violin

Some people say that everything the Robert Wood Johnson Foundation has done since day one has been aimed at improving health care quality. Indeed, one of the Foundation's initial three priorities, announced in 1972, was to improve the quality of health and medical care. Throughout the 1970s and 1980s, the Foundation financed a number of programs that could be considered to be directed at quality improvement, among them programs to improve quality of care offered at teaching hospitals, to develop tools to measure the quality of home health care, to help rural hospitals provide high-quality care, and to strengthen the quality of hospital nursing. But its efforts in the area were sporadic and largely unfocused.

The tempo picked up and the focus began to sharpen in the late 1980s and into the 1990s when the Foundation began awarding grants to build knowledge around the concept of quality—particularly, how to measure it. During this time, the Foundation supported studies by RAND's McGlynn on managed care's impact on mental health services and care for Medicare patients; Wennberg's *Dartmouth Atlas of Health Care*; and the Center for Studying Health System Change, which tracked how managed care was performing. The Foundation awarded grants to create the National Committee for Quality Assurance and the National Quality Forum—two organizations whose goal was to develop standards that would measure the quality of care provided by health plans and other providers.

The Foundation made important grants that were in fact directed toward improving quality, although they were not specifically denominated as such. These included grants to develop the chronic illness care model at Group Health Cooperative of Puget Sound, to strengthen hospital nursing, and to give terminally ill patients greater control of the care they receive toward the end of their lives.

During this time, staff members struggled to find ways for the Foundation to take on a greater role in quality. "Everything we were doing was quality but then nothing was," said Michael Rothman, who led the quality group when it was part of the Foundation's chronic illness care team. "We were working in areas that would improve quality, but we didn't phrase it that way," said Anne Weiss, who heads the Foundation's quality/equality team today. "When this got named—as it did with the *Quality Chasm* report—it was a signal that the problem was mature enough for us to take it on, as opposed to being a byproduct of things we were doing."

The difficulty, Rothman said, was that no one at the Foundation knew how to address quality. By the late 1990s, however, interest was building in adopting the science of quality improvement that had worked so well in companies such as Toyota and General Electric. These and other companies were using constant measurement and systematic organizational changes to improve their systems. They had remarkable success in eliminating defects, improving efficiency, and creating superior products.

Rothman brought to the Foundation the idea of supporting a project that had sprung up in Pittsburgh—led by Alcoa's chief (and later Treasury secretary) Paul O'Neill and Karen Wolk Feinstein, the president and chief executive officer of the Jewish Healthcare Foundation—to redesign health care by bringing in manufacturing methods such as Toyota's. The Foundation jumped on this idea and provided funds for Pittsburgh's effort in 2000. Over the following two years, the Foundation authorized another ambitious program that set out to transform American health care by using industry methods for achieving "perfection" and one that would test incentives for physicians and hospitals to provide better care to patients with chronic illnesses.

Looking back in 2006, Steven Schroeder, who headed the Foundation from 1990 to 2002, was startled to realize just how much quality work had been done under his leadership, although it had never been labeled as such. He concluded, "As I think back, we really did do a lot of work in quality. It was like a second violin—we weren't featuring it as a solo work."

The move from second to first chair of the violin section came when Risa Lavizzo-Mourey became Foundation president and chief executive officer in 2003. "Going forward, I wanted to emphasize quality improvement as something that people, both internally and externally, thought of the Foundation as doing," she said. For the first time, quality improvement became a strategic goal of the Foundation, which established a team focused exclusively on developing and monitoring programs in the area of quality.

In its work to improve quality, the Foundation has focused on five areas:

- Measuring the quality of care
- Reengineering hospitals and health systems
- Improving the working conditions of hospital nurses
- Changing the payment system to give incentives for care that meets quality standards
- Providing patient-centered care

A sixth area—reducing health disparities—was not initially considered to be part of the Foundation's "quality" portfolio, although staff members note that one of the goals of the Foundation's disparities work was to improve the quality of care received by racial and ethnic minorities. This would change later, and the Foundation's quality and disparities work would be integrated.

Measurement: The Beginning of Transparency and Accountability

A central tenet of the quality movement is that you can't fix what you can't measure, and in the early 1990s a push to develop standards against which you could measure the performance of health plans, hospitals, and doctors began to gain force. "You have to have standards that providers and health plans feel they have to live up to," said the former Robert Wood Johnson Foundation trustee Gail Warden.

The National Committee for Quality Assurance

Back in 1989, the managed care industry was exploding onto the national health care scene. There were about six hundred managed care plans, two-thirds of them not even five years old, with varying levels of quality and ability to assess and improve themselves. Health maintenance organizations had to meet federal qualification requirements related simply to the benefits they had to provide, not to quality or prevention services. Meanwhile, a skeptical public was concerned that the HMOs' drive to cut costs meant that their care would deteriorate.

In 1988, the Robert Wood Johnson Foundation gave a grant to an industry trade group to examine the feasibility of an accreditation program to certify managed care plans, with the certification based on standards of quality. The study concluded that such an organization could be created and would be useful in identifying the more and less worthy health plans.

In 1990, the trade group went independent as the nonprofit National Committee for Quality Assurance (NCQA), again with financial assistance from the Foundation. The time was right, said Margaret O'Kane, the founding and current president. "The HMOs were trying to figure out who they were, and were interested in cleaning up because there were some bad actors. This need converged with what was happening with employers, who were doing continuous quality improvement stuff in their businesses, understood the language of quality, and knew they weren't getting what they needed in health care."

NCQA conducted a survey of twenty-one managed care health plans in 1991, and in 1995 it began issuing a national report card. Meanwhile, a separate group of employers and some health plans were using the Health Plan Employer Data and Information Set (HEDIS), an evidence-based performance measurement tool that NCQA began to incorporate in 1992 and that has become the backbone of the NCQA accreditation program. With the HEDIS data standards, employers and consumers could compare the performance of various plans on such measures as annual mammograms for women once they reach fifty, childhood immunizations, measuring blood-sugar levels for diabetics, and giving beta blockers to people after a heart attack. By 1998, some 75 percent of people enrolled in managed care were in plans accredited by NCQA, and for its part, NCQA was able to show that its measuring of health plans had led to improvements in care.

The National Quality Forum

In 1998, recognizing that health care quality problems were not limited to managed care settings, President Clinton's Commission on Consumer Protection and Quality in the Health Care Industry issued a report, *Quality First,* that called for two organizations to be created to measure quality. One would be a private sector group—the National Quality Forum—that would standardize the many quality measures that were proliferating and publicly report them. The second organization would be a government entity to set goals and priorities for what would be measured, and to set the nation's agenda for quality improvement. While the NCQA measurements were to support a certification process for managed care plans, the National Quality Forum "is a much bigger effort," says Gail Warden, who was the founding board chair for the NCQA and then the National Quality Forum. "It reaches out further to all different members—researchers, providers, physicians, hospitals, and the ambulatory care community."

The National Quality Forum began operating in 1999, but the government body was never established, which led to what many critics describe as the Forum's unfulfilled promise in its early years. Set up as a membership organization composed of those with a stake in the measurements, the Forum was underfunded, and the measures it worked on were often determined by whichever group gave it financial support.

"Its organization and funding were such that it could only work on things it could get money for, so it was very opportunistic about what it could go for," said McGlynn, who also served on an early Forum strategy committee. "The membership approach led it to go after lowest-common-denominator measures. The impact was that it has been antagonistic to what I call 'best-in-class' measurement."

This was occurring at a time when many organizations were promoting their own standards. If you wanted to know the standard of care for, say, pain management, different measures might be available from a home health agency, a nursing home, and a hospital unit, not to mention an anesthesiologist society, a palliative care organization, and other groups. Instead of finding and promoting the one best measure, the National Quality Forum's measures simply added one more column of measures—adding to the cacophony, not reducing it as was intended.

The National Quality Forum's president, Janet Corrigan, agreed that the organization was not doing its intended job. In 2006, the Forum's board began what she called a "strategic repositioning." The Forum would now take on the annual priority-setting role that the government entity was to have had. It would work with all the interests—such as federal agencies, health plans, employers, unions, and consumer groups—to set national quality improvement standards. It would produce one common set of standards for everyone to use, and it would do this by putting out a call for measures in a particular area—such as breast cancer care—evaluating them all, and selecting the best one.

By deciding to develop its own priorities, Corrigan said, the organization hoped to zero in on areas that would make a substantial difference in the health of the largest number of patients. Corrigan also expected the Forum to develop process and outcome measures for how well patients fare with common chronic conditions over time. "I want to know how much better I will be if I manage this condition this way or that, and what is the difference in cost," said Corrigan. "That requires pulling lots of measures together and rolling them up into overall indicators."

In light of the National Quality Forum's reorganization and a $3 million Robert Wood Johnson Foundation grant in 2005 to further its work, many observers were optimistic that the Forum would achieve its main mission—giving the nation a common set of standards to evaluate health care quality.

Reengineering Health Care

The Pittsburgh Regional Health Initiative

Before the IOM reports on medical errors and quality, and before any hospitals started experimenting with industry engineering techniques to improve health care processes, a coalition of community leaders in Pittsburgh determined that the quality of health care in that city was unacceptable. They decided to use lessons that Toyota had implemented to make a product that was of higher quality and manufactured with efficiency methods that eliminated waste and respected workers' know-how. Their decision would be the start of a new way of thinking about how to cure what ails health care.

Leading the effort were Paul O'Neill and Karen Wolk Feinstein. Concerned about medical errors and care that fell way short of the mark, Feinstein sought out O'Neill, who had instituted policies that reduced injuries at Alcoa to almost zero. The company's culture had changed so much that even after O'Neill left, safety continued to improve.

Together they formed the Pittsburgh Regional Health Initiative, a coalition composed of chief executive officers from thirty hospitals (ten more would join later), health insurers, the attorney general (for antitrust issues), leaders of physician and nursing organizations, and business leaders. The two primary goals were to reduce hospital-acquired infections and medical errors that many in the health care industry believed were a given and probably impossible to eliminate.

"We were the first to say that pursuing anything short of perfection is a path to mediocrity," Feinstein said in an interview. "Aiming for mediocrity was what our current system was all about." The initiative introduced quality engineering principles that Alcoa had picked up from the Toyota Production System to redesign hospital processes in order to eliminate safety mistakes and become more efficient. Employees received training at Alcoa in this rigorous system, which the coalition called the Perfecting Patient Care System. Frontline hospital employees, working in teams, were empowered to structure their work for "continuous quality improvement." The quality innovation would emanate from the frontline workers who deliver patient care, and it would occur quickly, not after months of administrative reports and review. The health care teams would constantly assess how they were doing. In this way, the health care system would be redesigned to recognize and sweep out the stumbling blocks that caused mistakes.

Full disclosure of medical errors was critical to fixing processes that stood in the way of workers' giving patients the best care—but it was also a potential landmine if the media were to publicize the information. In a highly unusual move, the initiative reached an agreement with the city's two large newspapers not to practice "gotcha journalism" if performance reports were leaked to them that disclosed serious medical mistakes. The initiative promised that the bigger story, the transformation of a regional health system to eliminate danger to patients—the only such effort in the nation—would be a much better story. "We told them, 'If you publish the [performance] data, you will not have the story, because no one will want to participate with the initiative any more.' That would have undone the initiative," Feinstein said.

The Robert Wood Johnson Foundation provided $1 million toward Pittsburgh's effort from 2000 to 2003, which proved invaluable not just for the financial support but for the credibility it gave to this endeavor. The Foundation's funding attracted additional financial support from other sources.

The initiative dedicated itself to eradicating hospital-acquired central line–associated bloodstream infections that occur when a catheter spreads infection through the blood—a condition that causes many deaths. The thirty-two participating hospitals installed a database system for collecting information. Staff members rededicated themselves to making sure they did everything they knew they should do: they washed hands religiously, used gloves, covered themselves up appropriately, swabbed the area where the catheter was inserted, and avoided using several lines when possible. Mostly, the anti-infection campaign was about relentless attention to sanitation details.

The result? The infection rate was brought down an impressive 68 percent in four years. At Allegheny General Hospital, two intensive care units reduced central-line infections from forty-nine to six. Deaths from central line–associated infections dropped from nineteen to one over a year and remained negligible. Writing in the *The Joint Commission Journal on Quality and Patient Safety,* Dr. Rick Shannon of Allegheny General calculated that every central line-associated bloodstream infection averted saved the hospital nearly $27,000.[5]

The Veterans Health Administration's Pittsburgh Healthcare System in Pittsburgh mounted a campaign to stamp out antibiotic-resistant staph infection from its surgical units. A team scrubbed the clean equipment room and the supply room, placed gloves where they were easily accessible, and put signs to wash hands everywhere. "They did everything they could to eliminate pathways for infection," Feinstein said. "They would chart everything on the walls. Every day, they would measure progress to see if they were getting better or worse, to understand what drives infection transmission." The result? They lowered the staph infection rate by 85 percent.

The initiative ran into problems, however, with its goal to eliminate medication errors. The hospitals all used a new database to report errors in a reliable, consistent way, but they were frustrated by troubles in working with it. The largest hospital became preoccupied with other pressing computer matters. A plan to return illegible handwritten prescription orders to physicians fell through when doctors balked.

One discouraging lesson was that the commitment of hospital leaders was not sufficient to bring about wide use of the best practices that were developed. A hospital's top executives may be enthusiastic supporters, but they have to coordinate many competing interests such as physicians, insurers, boards of directors, employees, government and accreditation commission standards, and they need to make, not lose, money. "Quality is just there, floating with other everyday considerations that have to be balanced," Feinstein said. "They get rewarded for their bottom line. Quality leaders lose money because of the perverse payment system for coverage we have in this country, which actually rewards errors, because then you get paid for doing more."

Nevertheless, Pittsburgh made an impressive start, and it continued its quality improvement innovations after the Foundation's funding ended, taking redesign efforts to ambulatory care practices.

Pursuing Perfection and the 100,000 Lives Campaign

The Cincinnati Children's Hospital Medical Center's Cystic Fibrosis Center made a highly risky gesture when it invited parents to attend a meeting at which it would share lackluster performance data related to their children's health. Of the 116 cystic fibrosis centers across the nation, Cincinnati Children's was just "in the middle of the pack" when it came to its young patients' lung functioning, and about 40 percent of the children's weights—a major indicator of how they were doing—were beneath the tenth percentile for their ages. These two factors are predictors of how long children with this disease, whose average lifespan is thirty-three years, can be expected to live.

Although the parents were disheartened to learn that the care their children were receiving was merely average, they were impressed with the center's openness and honesty. So when the hospital asked them to help redesign the system to improve care, they signed on and began sharing ideas and concerns. At first, they divided into two groups—the staff would come up with what it believed were the families' top ten priorities for change, and the families would do the same for the staff. Instructively, the providers' list showed that they often didn't know what the families felt they needed, said Tracey Blackwelder, an active family participant with four children treated at the center. For instance, the providers believed that reducing wait times in the clinic would be a top priority to parents, but they said no, getting all their needs met at the clinic visit was far more important. So, together with the providers, the families developed a questionnaire that is sent to them two weeks before a visit; in it they note their concerns, the questions they need answered, and any specialists they need to see. Doctors then structure the clinic visits to meet those needs. "Now when families come in, the doctor is prepared to answer their concerns," Blackwelder said. "This has helped us all to work together as a team."

The Center took steps to work more rigorously to improve the kids' lung function and nutritional status: taking respiratory cultures every three months and closely monitoring the kids' weight and height, so that measures could be taken early to stop downward spirals. "Height and weight was one area that was very important to parents, and we worked on it a long time," Blackwelder said. "We made sure any kid under the tenth percentile for height and weight was given a kind of red flag—it was a goal that no one would be in the tenth percentile." The nutritionist would chart monthly results, and all would cheer as kids made it out of the tenth percentile. "To see this work was pretty cool," Blackwelder said. Parents also pushed for all kids to be given flu shots to prevent secondary respiratory infections, and parents and doctors kept an eye on innovations at other cystic fibrosis centers to learn the fine points of what was working well elsewhere.

This intensive effort brought the intended results. Fewer than 25 percent of the patients are now in the very low weight category. Eighty-five percent of the children have a quarterly respiratory culture; three years ago, just 50 percent had them. Flu shots are given to more than 95 percent of the kids, up from 40 percent before this effort began. Meanwhile, Cincinnati Children's learned a major lesson: parent involvement and being open about how it was performing—transparency—were vital to what the center was about.

"The parents changed everything for us," said Uma Kotagal, Cincinnati Children's senior vice president for quality and transformation, who headed the hospital's efforts under the Robert Wood Johnson Foundation grant Pursuing Perfection: Raising the Bar for Health Care Performance. (The Cystic Fibrosis Center was but one piece of the hospital's program.) "They are the real experts when it comes to their children."

Cincinnati Children's was one of seven locations to take part in the Foundation's Pursuing Perfection initiative, an eight-year, $26 million program initially funded in and managed by the Institute for Healthcare Improvement.[6] This program was a response to the IOM's two reports,

To Err Is Human and *Crossing the Quality Chasm*; the Institute of Healthcare Improvement president, Donald Berwick, had a major hand in drafting its executive summary. Pursuing Perfection took the report's blueprint for redesigning the care processes as its own—insisting on care that was safe, effective, patient-centered, timely, efficient, and equitable. It also drew from the Pittsburgh Regional Health Initiative, a "very helpful prototype," according to Berwick.

Pursuing Perfection aimed at creating one or more models of ways to transform health care—or create a new "Toyota" model for redesigning health care. It used industry methods to improve patients' health outcomes by changing the patient care processes. It insisted that hospitals' troubles were systemic and that blame for them could not be placed at the feet of workers who were burdened by a broken system. To improve outcomes, it sought to change patient care systems. Simply achieving benchmarks for average performance wouldn't be adequate anymore; Pursuing Perfection hospitals would aim for perfection.

Industry methods included "continuous quality improvement" and "rapid cycles of change." As with Pittsburgh, frontline employees were empowered to constantly assess their processes, suggest innovations, implement those that were improvements, and monitor how they worked out. The program also borrowed from the Six Sigma approach used at Motorola and General Electric, with its emphasis on rooting out defects. The seven sites applied evidence-based medicine to ensure that all patients benefited from high standards, but they customized care for some whose cases were more complex or unusual and needed different approaches.

All of the hospitals made great strides in improvement, and some came close to transformation, especially Cincinnati Children's. Here is a sampling:

- Tallahassee Memorial Health Care wanted to find out why its death rates were well above the national average. As a Pursuing Perfection grantee, it examined the hospital's death records and found a number of contributing factors: not noticing when a patient was deteriorating and needed quick intervention, communication failures such as between providers and nurses or between a patient and a nurse, and deficiencies in the patient's diagnosis and treatment. The Institute for Healthcare Improvement suggested a number of strategies that Tallahassee adopted. It created, for example, rapid response teams to provide nurses with the resources they needed when they sensed a patient's condition was quickly worsening, and "multidisciplinary rounds" with a physician, a nurse, a pharmacist, and a therapist to improve patients' communication and care planning. The upshot? Deaths were reduced by almost 31 percent between 2001 and 2004. This translated to 53 percent fewer deaths from acute myocardial infarction, 62 percent fewer from heart failure, 41 percent fewer from stroke, and 46 percent fewer from pneumonia.

- At McLeod Regional Medical Center in Florence, South Carolina, the medication error rate was at the low end of the national average, but leaders there felt that it could be far better. McLeod set a goal of zero drug mistakes. It created teams to make plans to improve medication safety. More doctors began using handheld computers to track drugs. Medications whose names look and sound alike were separated on carts. Top administrators toured the floors daily, asking staff about impediments to medication safety. The hospital bought a computerized drug-ordering system, which spots a patient's possible medication interactions and eliminates one fertile spot for errors: the handwritten prescription order. And it instituted a "medication administration checker" that scans bar codes on a patient's armband and the medication to confirm that this is the proper drug and in the proper amount before it is given. The outcome? The number of adverse drug events declined from more than two for every one thousand doses in 2002 to less than one per one thousand in the first half of 2004.

- Hackensack University Medical Center in Hackensack, New Jersey, is known as one of the best hospitals in the country for cardiac care, but it wanted to become even better. Among other things, the hospital speeded up processes and added safeguards to ensure that no necessary care step was forgotten. The emergency department coordinated care with paramedics, who ran EKGs on the patient in the ambulance, sending results ahead. Nurses received more training on how best to tend to patients having heart attacks. For example, if the EKG indicated certain specified warning signs, the catheterization lab and a cardiologist were notified immediately, and an emergency department nurse gave the patient aspirin and beta blockers and rushed him or her to the catheterization lab. The result? Death from acute myocardial infarction was lowered to about 5 percent, well below the 10.9 percent national average.

Although much was learned in Pursuing Perfection, and the sites showed how to accelerate the pace of change, as had been hoped, the biggest goal was not achieved. "The bottom line, of course, is this: We do not have a Toyota in health care," wrote Berwick, along with the executive director of the Institute for Healthcare Improvement, Andrea Kabcenell, and Thomas Nolan, an Institute senior fellow, in an article for *Modern Healthcare.* "The project's primary goal—total system transformation with unprecedented total performance—remains, frankly to no one's surprise, still out of reach. But it is no longer out of sight. The progress has been extraordinary."[7] Berwick himself, although pleased with the overall effort, faulted the program for not working seriously with hospital financial officers on the basic monetary issues that can hinder quality improvement. "We dropped the ball on the financial case," he said.

Many of the lessons from Pursuing Perfection were used in the Institute for Healthcare Improvement's learning collaboratives and became resources on the Institute's Web site. They were also keys to the 100,000 Lives Campaign, a highly publicized effort to prevent medical errors in the more than three thousand hospitals that adopted evidence-based strategies such as giving beta blockers and aspirin to heart attack victims; using rapid-response teams for medical crises; and checking at each juncture to be sure that the correct medications were being given to patients. The campaign attracted widespread media attention when it announced that it had saved more than 122,000 lives over eighteen months.

Although experts raised probing questions about how the campaign arrived at the number of saved lives and the initiative's assumption that rapid-response teams were a best practice, the campaign was largely viewed as a victory for quality improvement. "This is the most thrilling episode in my whole career," Berwick said in an interview. "It showed it could be done." In late 2006, his institute expanded on the momentum from the 100,000 Lives campaign by announcing the 5 Million Lives Campaign, which would work to prevent five million injuries from causes such as bedsores, drug-resistant staph infections, and congestive heart failure.

Nursing: Transforming Care at the Bedside

Like nearly all hospitals, says nurse Millicent De Jesus, her general surgical unit at Cedars-Sinai Medical Center in Los Angeles has had its "fair share of medication errors." The nurses in the unit felt they knew why: they prepared each patient's medications at the nursing station, where doctors, patients, and family members constantly interrupted and distracted them. So when the nurses' station was being redesigned and their input was solicited, the nurses came up with the idea of creating a separate medication room where they wouldn't be disturbed. And they gave a lot of suggestions about what would make the perfect medication room. The idea was turned into a reality, and it's called the "no-interrupt zone." "The nurses were very happy because they had a say, they were involved in how they would like our environment changed and processes improved," De Jesus said.

De Jesus's forty-eight-bed general surgery unit is one of the success stories to emerge from Transforming Care at the Bedside, another Foundation-funded initiative that is managed by the Institute for Healthcare Improvement. Begun in 2003 as a pilot with three hospitals that tried out concepts, it expanded in 2004 to seventeen medical-surgical units in hospitals around the nation.

Transforming Care at the Bedside was designed to address the nation's pressing nursing shortage and tie it into the Foundation's focus on improving the quality of health care. It targeted what much research has shown to be the underlying reason that people were either not attracted to nursing or leaving it in droves—the poor working environment. Nurses put it this way: they spend too much time on paperwork and hunting down equipment all over the hospital; physicians are rude and disrespectful to them; they have little autonomy; and they're given little support when the workload gets stressful. Finally, they don't have enough time to do the job they were trained for—taking care of patients.

"We wanted to do what we could to change the work environment to make nurses excited about the work they do," said Susan Hassmiller, the Robert Wood Johnson Foundation's senior program officer who oversees Transforming Care and is herself a nurse. "We believed that if we could get more nurses really engaged and excited about the care that they give, they would stay and give a better quality of care. It's not really brain surgery."

The Transforming Care at the Bedside units started their work with what is called a *brainstorming deep dive,* with frontline nurses sitting in a room, thinking about the care they provide and the countless processes behind the care, and considering what they could improve in their work environment and patient care. (Later, they would regularly do smaller dives, which they called *snorkels.*) The innovations they came up with out of this brainstorming were always in one of four areas of focus: reliability, getting the waste out of work processes, patient centeredness, and increasing nurse vitality. Worthy ideas were tested quickly and then "adopted, adapted, or abandoned," in the lingo of the program.

The top priority for the nurses in the units was increasing their time by the patient's side. Nationally, hospital nurses spend an average of about 35 percent of their time with patients; the program set a goal of 70 percent at the bedside. "How does this goal tie into quality?" Hassmiller asked. "If the nurse is not in the room observing a patient's color, activity, smell, and sounds, something bad could happen. You will have a patient falling, having adverse effects, developing bedsores."

Transforming Care at the Bedside emphasizes a bottom-up approach, with nurses who deliver patient care devising better ways to do things. This requires support of the nurses' ideas by both the hospital's administrators and its middle managers. The bread and butter of the program is identifying small changes that make a big difference. Here are some of the modest proposals nurses have come up with:

- Put look-alike, sound-alike medications on separate carts
- Create "lift teams" that help nurses if they have a patient who needs to be turned or lifted—thereby preventing injuries that commonly plague nurses
- Move some supplies such as linens into patients' rooms instead of keeping them in supply cabinets on the floor

- Assign nurses to specialize in admissions so that other nurses aren't distracted by the need to suddenly admit a new patient
- Reduce paperwork requirements

At Los Angeles' Cedars-Sinai, nurses now accompany physicians on rounds. Doctors had always resisted this at Cedars-Sinai because they believed that having a nurse with them would take up too much time, said Peachy Hain, who heads the Cedars-Sinai Transforming Care unit where De Jesus works. "We told the doctors, 'We have to call you ten times during the day because we can't read your orders and we can't read your mind. If we're there with you on rounds, we won't be bothering you the rest of the day.'" Walking rounds and reviewing each patient's care plan together led to more courtesy, respect, and teamwork among doctors and nurses—and improved the nurses' enthusiasm for the job. "The doctors don't get angry at the nurses anymore because of that camaraderie they developed constantly walking rounds, planning care together, coordinating what needs to be done for the patient," Hain said.

At the Cedars-Sinai unit, the amount of time lost to paperwork has gone down from 30 percent to 7 percent. The nurses designed a "patient care pack" that outlines what patients need to know about their stay. In the patient's progress notes, the nurse is now able to write, "progressing per patient care pack," instead of repeatedly writing the same notes for each patient. They jot down only what is abnormal or a point that wasn't in the care pack. "It helps when you have an environment where nurses feel there's a better future not just for patients but for the staff because they're being listened to and appreciated," Hain said.

The program is currently being evaluated by a team from the University of California, Los Angeles, and RAND Health. According to the leader of the evaluation team, Jack Needleman of UCLA, preliminary data show that voluntary departures by nurses from Transforming Care at the Bedside units have declined and that some units that have had difficulty recruiting in the past are reporting waiting lists for positions. The units are testing, on average, one innovation per month. As a result of this work, nurses on the Transforming Care at the Bedside units are spending more than half their time in direct patient care, with one hospital, Cedars-Sinai, increasing the percentage of time in direct patient care from 47 percent in the first six months of the program to 71 percent in the last six months it reported.

Rewarding Results, or Experiments in Pay for Performance

The nation's irrational payment system rewards health care providers for mistakes. Healthier patients mean fewer occupied beds and less revenue for hospitals. If the wrong kidney is removed from a patient, the surgeon and the hospital make more money out of correcting the tragic mistake than if the correct kidney had been taken out. A physician who decides to manage his diabetic patients more aggressively with more tracking of tests, e-mail and telephone consultations, and ongoing educational assistance about lifestyle adjustments will likely find that patients have fewer complications and thus fewer office visits and hospitalizations. He or she can lose money by providing quality care that insurance doesn't cover.

Awareness of the need to reform these distorted incentives led in the early 2000s to increased interest in a "pay for performance" (P4P) approach that would reward providers for care that met certain best-practice standards. In 2002, the Robert Wood Johnson Foundation, together with the California HealthCare Foundation, kicked off an initiative—Rewarding Results: Aligning Incentives with High-Quality Health Care—to test a range of P4P approaches. This five-year, $8.9 million program was also supported by the Commonwealth Fund and managed by the Leapfrog Group in Washington, D.C., which was founded by Fortune 500 and government purchasers of health care hoping to bring accountability to health care.

Seven organizations—five funded by the Robert Wood Johnson Foundation and two by the California Healthcare Foundation—were selected to run demonstration projects: Blue Cross Blue Shield of Michigan, Blue Cross of California, Bridges to Excellence, the Excellus Health Plan/Rochester Individual Practice Association, the Integrated Healthcare Association, Local Initiative Rewarding Results (for babies and teenagers covered by Medicaid), and Massachusetts Health Quality Partners. The idea was to provide incentives for quality and investing in the expensive infrastructure needed to help improve quality. The seven Rewarding Results projects would set goals for achieving certain best practices, evaluate performance, make these measures public, and reward providers for providing appropriate care. The program used a broad range of strategies, such as making bonus payments for reaching specified performance goals (for example, hemoglobin A1c testing for people with diabetes), providing educational benefits, and helping doctors with the cost of installing information technology.

"P4P is meant to encourage providers to get systems in place and implement best practices," said Leapfrog's chief operating officer, Karen Linscott. "We have to get current best practice incorporated into everyday practice, but that can take up to seventeen years. We think incentives can help to motivate providers to decide to move more quickly."

One example of how the program works is Bridges to Excellence. The coalition collaborated with the National Committee for Quality Assurance to develop best-practices standards for treating diabetic patients (such as checking kidney function, feet, eyes, and blood-sugar levels), and started using them in three cities: Boston, Cincinnati, and Louisville, Kentucky. Physician groups that met those standards were eligible for a bonus. The incentive apparently worked; Bridges to Excellence doctors were able to see twice as many diabetic patients as they had before, and costs declined 15 to 20 percent.

"These projects add to the mounting evidence that rewarding good performance can encourage doctors to provide appropriate care to patients to help them live longer and healthier lives," said Karen Davis, president of the Commonwealth Fund. Even so, the approach has its critics. They question whether doctors will, in effect, be penalized if their patients don't follow through on quality measures—don't have bloodwork done, for example—or whether P4P will hamstring doctors by forcing them to stick to guidelines and not strive to find better solutions for their patients.

Suzanne Delbanco, Leapfrog's chief executive officer, observed that the demonstration projects, although far from conclusive, provided "some of the first tangible evidence that P4P incentives can raise the quality of patient care." She cautions that it is still too soon to endorse P4P and that more assessment is needed. Leapfrog's materials caution that P4P "is not a magic bullet," but just one of many efforts to try to address the need for better incentives in financing medical care.

To most observers, Rewarding Results—along with the similar experiments funded by the federal Agency for Healthcare Research and Quality and the Centers for Medicare & Medicaid Services—contributed some knowledge to the debate and amounted to a first stage of learning about P4P. As of the end of 2006, P4P took on even more importance, with the Centers for Medicare & Medicaid Services' announcement of 1.5 percent bonuses to physicians who report their performance on certain quality standards.

Patient-Centered Care

With nearly three-quarters of health care spending now going toward chronic illness care, the need to figure out how to get patients engaged in their own care—even shaping it—has become critical. The IOM's *Quality Chasm* report declared that in the redesign of the health care system, patient-centered care and patient self-management should play major roles. This is a fundamentally different approach to patient care than the traditional one. It signifies a collaborative effort between patients and physicians (and their health care team). For their part, patients—especially those with chronic conditions—must play a role in managing their illness by taking their medications, eating properly, exercising, and doing those things that will maintain their health. For physicians and their teams, it means taking time to understand their patients, educate them, and help them through whatever prevents them from following a healthful regimen.

Besides the patient-centered aspects of the Pursuing Perfection grants, the Robert Wood Johnson Foundation supported a number of efforts intended to help promote progress in patient-centered care, some of which are described below.

Quality Allies/New Health Partnerships

Quality Allies: Improving Care by Engaging Patients is a $3.50 million, three-year initiative, cofunded with the California HealthCare Foundation and managed by the Institute for Healthcare Improvement, to help outpatient providers develop effective collaborative approaches to working with patients and their families to support them in self-managing a chronic condition. In an earlier companion pilot program, six provider teams, along with expert faculty, developed a curriculum to help guide the way self-management support could be given. It entails providers talking to patients about their interests, values, and preferences in a way that encourages them to become engaged in planning their own care. Providers then must follow up with patients to see if the plan meets their needs or requires tweaking.

"Self-management support tends to be the main driver in being able to achieve high-quality outcomes and process measures for people with chronic health conditions," said Doriane Miller, a physician and former Foundation vice president, who directs Quality Allies. "But in some medical circles this could be considered heretical, in that the doctor is always right and patients come to the doctor as a learned adviser, not as a collaborator."

In 2005, twenty practitioner teams from around the nation were chosen to work for one year on collaborative self-management projects of their choosing, applying concepts developed in the pilots. Each team had to have a patient and a family member as an active planner of the project to gain the patient perspective.

For example, Harlem Hospital in New York City helped people with HIV follow medication recommendations and keep doctor appointments. A Santa Clara Valley Medical Center team in California developed better outreach and support for people with depression. A multiple sclerosis clinic at the Medical College of Georgia found ways to teach patients to use an online self-management support Web site so their doctor could help them manage their symptoms. In Fargo, North Dakota, an online portal was set up for people with diabetes to talk with one another about their medical problems and concerns, gain support, and create a sense of community.

Patients and family members have reacted well to Quality Allies, and processes of care for self-management have improved, Miller said. She noted that in some cases, the teams were able to help health plans and providers make a business case that by improving their care systems, they were better able to meet HEDIS care indicators—and could negotiate a higher rate of reimbursement for their services. Whether these sites will be able to sustain changes for the people who participated is yet to be determined.

The Quality Allies program, which was absorbed into another Institute for Healthcare Improvement program called New Health Partnerships, turned to its next phase—a distance learning program—in March of 2007. New Health Partnerships allows for the transfer of knowledge gained from the demonstration projects to a wide audience on the Web. New Health Partnerships set up two Web sites, one offering information and interaction for patients and families, the other providing a broad array of assistance for physicians. "We've had twenty-six organizations that have had face-to-face demonstrations," Miller said. "There is a need for this to spread in a practical way. Demonstrations are labor-intensive and costly and not as efficient in terms of making sure we get widespread changes."

Developing a Patient-Activation Measure

The Foundation also funded research that led to the creation of a "patient activation measure" by Judith Hibbard, a professor at the University of Oregon and noted quality expert. She developed the measure to predict how people with chronic conditions can be expected to behave—from doing healthy things for themselves to managing specific diseases to preventive efforts such as using quality information.

The answers to the thirteen questions in the patient-activation measure can predict the degree to which people have the ability and the confidence to manage their own health and health care. It can predict, for example, whether someone probably will or won't take medications and exercise if told to. Hibbard's research has identified four stages on a person's way to becoming a competent self-manager. Using the patient-activation measure will help physicians and their teams customize their approach to involving patients in their own care. "It's really about using this as a guide to think about the challenges people face at each of the stages," Hibbard said.

Advocacy

In another patient-centered grant, the National Partnership for Women & Families is marshalling consumer and patient advocacy groups to become a stronger voice for changes to the health care system that will improve the quality of care. Begun in 2004, the program reaches out to local grassroots organizations as well as national advocacy groups. The partnership gives technical assistance to local groups, such as Easter Seals chapters and local clubs, helping them understand how the current debate on health care quality improvement affects them and how to become engaged participants. On the national level, the partnership works with groups such as the AFL-CIO, Consumers Union, and the National Coalition for Cancer Survivorship to make sure that their efforts of quality and transparency meet consumer needs. Measurement, for example, is an important issue for consumers but often falls short of what they need. "We push the envelope and get to measures that will help us better understand outcomes," said Debra Ness, president of the partnership. "There are a lot of measures that would be more meaningful to consumers than what we now have. That's why consumers have to make sure they have a voice."

The Next Steps: Linking Quality and Equality

By 2005, many of the strands of the Robert Wood Johnson Foundation's work to improve quality of care were coming together. Through its work with the National Committee on Quality Assurance, the National Quality Forum, and other groups, the Foundation had assisted in the establishment of standards against which businesses and the public could measure the performance of health plans, hospitals, and physicians. It had funded the development and expansion of the chronic care model, which became a key component in the delivery of high-quality care to chronically ill people and a basis of pay-for-performance incentives. It had financed approaches in Pittsburgh and elsewhere that brought modern business practices to health care, including nursing care. Its support of palliative care had given dying patients and their families a greater say in the kind of care they chose to receive, and it had supported other efforts to make health care more of a joint effort involving patients and health care professionals.

The next step was to weave the strands into a tapestry that would enable communities to quicken the pace of improvement and do so on a larger scale than they otherwise could have. The Foundation decided to do this initially through a strategy focused on regional health care markets. In 2005, the Foundation launched Aligning Forces for Quality: The Regional Market Project. A $14 million program managed by the Center for Health Improvement in Sacramento, it awarded grants to fourteen communitywide coalitions of local stakeholders—physicians, insurers, hospitals, employers, and consumers. They are bundling three important components of quality: (1) enhancing transparency by measuring and publicly reporting on local physicians' performance, (2) creating the local infrastructure to help physicians improve their outpatient care, and (3) generating consumer engagement by using quality measures to choose high-performing providers.

"We're trying to break down the silos of the stakeholder organizations and meet our three aims," said Gregg Shibata, the center's associate director. "We want there to be no line separating quality improvement and transparency, and no line between consumer engagement efforts and transparency."

Even as Aligning Forces was getting underway, the Foundation's board of trustees took a dramatic step. In 2006, it decided to consolidate the Foundation's grantmaking into a single priority area to improve quality and to decrease disparities.

For many years, the Foundation had financed projects whose goal was to reduce disparities in health—and in access to quality health care—between disadvantaged minorities and whites. Minorities have higher rates than whites of cardiovascular disease, diabetes, some cancers, obesity, and many other illnesses and unhealthy conditions. Many of the programs to reduce disparities involved research, but others attempted to improve the care received by African Americans, Latinos, and other ethnic minorities.

In combining its quality and disparities programming, the Foundation brought together its work in both areas. The new strategic priority area is called *quality/equality.* Very quickly, the Foundation's quality/equality team began to consider how to apply the tools of quality improvement to the challenge of health care disparities.

An example of the kind of programs the Foundation plans to support under the quality/equality rubric is Expecting Success: Excellence in Cardiac Care, a four-year, $13 million initiative involving ten hospitals that the Foundation authorized in 2004. The program is focused on ensuring that African Americans, Latinos, and other minorities receive the same standard of quality care for cardiovascular disease that whites receive—for example, receiving beta blockers in the event of a heart attack. All of the grantee hospitals, which have formed a collaborative to learn from each other, are also encouraging quality cardiac prevention and care in the surrounding communities.

End Note

In recent years, Donald Berwick and a host of other leaders of the quality movement have spearheaded progress toward redesigning the array of systems that make up American health care. By 2007, the first stage of the quality improvement movement was ending, with advances achieved in setting measurable standards for performance, reengineering hospitals to make quality and safety top priorities, exploring pay for performance, and finding ways to put patients at the center of their own health care. Although these changes have not been widely adopted throughout the country and the insurance system remains skewed toward reimbursing costly, high-tech curative care, they are being followed in a number of places.

The Foundation has acted as something of a midwife to this movement, providing the financial support and influence to help most of the major players carry out much of the early important research, experiments, and demonstrations on quality. Its resources have been directed at many separate aspects of the problem, but an overarching approach that brings all of the forces together appears to hold the most promise.

Now this movement heads into its next phase. For many of those involved it is like remodeling a house while still living in it—they are antsy, impatient, and sometimes don't see much progress or are disappointed by setbacks. But there is recognition, too, when all is said and done, that signs of change are adding up and there's much to cheer about—from the development of quality improvement leadership to a recognition of what the problems are and from doctors' offices with new information technology systems to health plans that have begun to inject quality measures into their payment reimbursements.

"We have managed over the last few years to break down a lot of myths about how health care can't get any better, that it's just the way it is, [that] there are always going to be errors," said the National Quality Forum's Janet Corrigan. "People realize now that it doesn't have to be this way. We can make it a whole lot better."

Notes

1. Newbergh, C. "The Dartmouth Atlas of Healthcare." In *To Improve Health and Health Care, Volume XI: The Robert Wood Johnson Foundation Anthology.* San Francisco: Jossey-Bass, 2006.
2. Institute of Medicine. *To Err Is Human: Building a Safer Health System.* Washington, D.C.: National Academies Press, 2000.
3. Institute of Medicine. *Crossing the Quality Chasm: A New Health System for the 21st Century.* Washington, D.C.: National Academies Press, 2001.
4. McGlynn, E. A., and others. "The Quality of Health Care Delivered to Adults in the United States." *New England Journal of Medicine,* 2003, *348*(26), 2635–2645.
5. Gardner, J. R., and Harrison, A. R. "The Robert Wood Johnson Foundation: The Early Years." In *To Improve Health and Health Care, Vol. VIII The Robert Wood Johnson Foundation Anthology.* San Francisco: Jossey-Bass, 2005.
6. The Robert Wood Johnson Foundation. Topic Summary: RWJF's Strategy and Direction to Improve Health Care Quality 1972 to 2006. (http://www.rwjf.org/files/publications/other/HealthcareQualityReport_041207.pdf?gsa=1)
7. Shannon, R. B., and others. "Using Real-Time Problem Solving to Eliminate Central Line Infections." *Joint Commission Journal on Quality and Patient Safety,* 2006, *32*(9), 479–487.
8. In addition to the seven sites funded by the Robert Wood Johnson Foundation, the Institute for Healthcare Improvement had six more sites in the United States and Europe.
9. Berwick, D., Kabcenell, A., and Nolan, T. "Pursuing Perfection: No Toyota Yet, But a Start." *Modern Healthcare,* Sept. 26, 2006.

CHAPTER 2

Health Services Research

David C. Colby

Editor's Introduction

Among the strategies employed by the Robert Wood Johnson Foundation is the creation and nurturing of new fields.[1] In the 1970s and 1980s, the Foundation funded the development of a new field of health care professionals—nurse practitioners.[2] In the 1990s, it seeded and supported the new field of tobacco-policy research.[3] That same decade, the Foundation's funding, along with that of the Open Society Institute, advanced the field of palliative care.[4] As discussed in Chapter One of this volume, the Foundation has also been influential in developing quality of care as a field.[5]

In this chapter, David Colby examines the Foundation's role in creating the field of health services research. As Colby, the Foundation's vice president for research and evaluation (and coeditor of this volume), describes it, building the field came about as a byproduct of the Foundation's support of research and researchers that could help the Foundation improve its own programming efforts. It was only late in the game that Foundation officials realized that they had created what could be considered a field and began providing core support to two of its main pillars: AcademyHealth, the organization that serves as the hub of the health services researchers' network, and *Health Affairs,* the field's premier research and policy journal. However circuitous the way of getting there, health services research is now a vibrant and well-respected academic field.

David Colby, in addition to serving as a Foundation interim vice president, is himself a noted health services research and policy expert. Before joining the Robert Wood Johnson Foundation, he was a Robert Wood Johnson Faculty Fellow in Health Care Finance, an associate editor of the *Journal of Health Politics, Policy and Law,* a member of the faculty of the University of Maryland Baltimore County, and a staff member of the Physician Payment Review Commission and the Medicare Payment Advisory Commission.

S.L.I.

Notes

1. Isaacs, S. L., and Knickman, J. R. "Field Building: Lessons from the Robert Wood Johnson Foundation's Anthology Series." *Health Affairs,* 2005, *24*(4), 1161–1165.
2. Kennan, T. "In Support of Nurse Practitioners and Physician Assistants." *To Improve Health and Health Care, 1988–1989: The Robert Wood Johnson Foundation Anthology.* San Francisco: Jossey-Bass, 1989
3. Warner, K. E. "Tobacco Policy Research: Insights and Contributions to Public Health Policy." *Tobacco Control Policy.* San Francisco: Jossey-Bass, 2006.
4. Bronner, E. "End-of-Life Programs." *To Improve Health and Health Care, Vol. VI: The Robert Wood Johnson Foundation Anthology.* San Francisco: Jossey-Bass, 2003.
5. See Chapter One in this volume.

In the days when health care was little more than a cottage industry, with only a slight impact on the economy, interest in studying it was limited. Many people can claim some part in the creation of what is now known as "health services research." One of them was Ernest Codman, a physician who, in the 1910s, classified hospital discharges, the number of medical errors, and the reasons for those errors. Other pioneers include Harry Moore, an economist with the United States Public Health Service, and I. S. Falk, a medical researcher and professor at the University of Chicago, who, in the late 1920s and the early 1930s, provided broad-ranging socioeconomic research for the influential Committee on the Cost of Medical Care. In the 1950s, Milton Roemer, a physician at the UCLA School of Public Health, conducted pathbreaking research, including an eponymous law that "a bed built is a bed filled," meaning that the supply of hospital beds determined the demand for hospital services. In 1964, the health maintenance organization Kaiser Permanente hired Merwyn Greenlick, an expert in the organization of medical care, as director of what was to become its Center for Health Services Research. In that position, Greenlick became a leader in health services research, conducting demonstrations including ones on prospective payment for Medicare services and the use of social health maintenance organizations to provide social and medical services for frail elders.

In the 1960s, "health services research" became recognized as an academic discipline in its own right. As the influential Columbia University economist Eli Ginzberg noted, the passage of Medicare and Medicaid in the mid-1960s, with the ensuing increase in health care costs, was the turning point in the development and support of health services research.[1] According to Lawrence Brown, a professor of health policy at the Mailman School of Public Health of Columbia University, from 1964 on the United States government funded studies of the demand and supply of

---

The author thanks Linda Aiken, Bob Blendon, Alan Cohen, Anne Gauthier, David Helms, and John Iglehart for their valuable insights. Special thanks to Melanie Napier for research assistance.

health services to understand what was driving inflation in the health care system.[2]

The 1960s saw the establishment of organizations and professional journals dedicated to health services research. The journals *Medical Care, Inquiry,* and *Health Services Research* were founded in the 1960s. The Medical Care Section of the American Public Health Association was founded in 1963. In 1968, the first formal federal support for the field came through the establishment of the National Center for Health Services Research and Development, a forerunner of the Agency for Healthcare Research and Quality. The field, however, did not form its own professional organization, the Association for Health Services Research (now known as AcademyHealth) until 1981.

In the half-century since the initial publication of *Medical Care,* health services research has grown into an important academic field, albeit one whose boundaries are somewhat fuzzy. The Institute of Medicine defines health services research as "a multidisciplinary field of inquiry, both basic and applied, that examines the use, costs, quality, accessibility, delivery, organization, financing, and outcomes of health care services to increase knowledge and understanding of the structure, processes, and effects of health services for individuals and populations."[3] Health services research is funded by the government (primarily through the Agency for Healthcare Quality and Research, the National Institutes of Health, and the Centers for Medicare & Medicaid Services) and by foundations (most visibly the Robert Wood Johnson Foundation, the Commonwealth Fund, the California HealthCare Foundation, and the Henry J. Kaiser Family Foundation). Today more than thirty American universities award doctorates in public health with an emphasis on health services research, and AcademyHealth boasts a membership of approximately four thousand health services researchers.

Since its earliest days, the Robert Wood Johnson Foundation has been influential in creating and advancing the field of health services research. To do this, it adopted three approaches: supporting research and its dissemination, developing a core of health services researchers, and strengthening organizations in the field. In the early years, however, the Foundation's support of health service research included only the first two of these approaches. Support of health services research as a field came much later.

The Foundation's Approach in the Early Years (1972–1976)

During the Foundation's early years, its founding staff and board members felt that they were seeing the culmination of a forty-year debate over the need to eliminate economic barriers to access to health care. They expected that by 1975 the nation would adopt national health insurance and thought that within that context, the Foundation had a unique opportunity to reshape the structure of health care delivery.

What role would research play in this effort? The intention was to fund and to be a consumer of research that would further the Foundation's mission; there was no intention of building a field at that time. The staff and the board saw the Foundation's research as "mission-oriented"; that is, the Foundation was not interested in funding health services research just for the sake of research or for more theoretical reasons. This has always been the justification for funding of research at the Foundation.

Given this mission-oriented approach, the Foundation's board and staff members were interested primarily in research that examined problems that concerned them and that provided information for new programs. For example, because they were interested in access to care, they funded surveys to find out where people went to obtain medical care. Second, they funded studies evaluating the Foundation's programs. The 1973 *Annual Report* noted that the Foundation would develop demonstration programs, evaluate them, and provide information to others. They felt that the spread of interventions required "solid objective data."[4]

In addition, the Foundation decided to support health policy analysis. In 1973, it funded the Health Policy Program at the University of California, San Francisco, headed by Philip Lee (former assistant secretary of the Department of Health, Education and Welfare), to conduct policy analysis and to train students in policy research. Later, this program became the Institute for Health Policy Studies, a major center for health services research.[5]

Thus, most of the early health services research to identify problems and evaluate programs was highly directed: staff members knew what information they wanted and then found the person they felt would do the best job of conducting the research and disseminating the results.

The exception to this directed research was the "great men awards"—research initiated by eminent researchers, selected on the basis of their stature, that explored topics that could help the Foundation identify areas for its future work. The "great men" had a permissive set of ground rules that allowed them creativity and wide-ranging explorations. Among the recipients of these awards were the City College of New York and later Stanford University economist Victor Fuchs, who from 1973 to 1988 examined, among other topics, the economic measurement of health, the cost of health care, national health insurance, and improving health markets; David Mechanic, a sociologist at the University of Wisconsin and later at Rutgers, who from 1973 to 1987 researched the organization of medical care; Eli Ginzberg, who worked on health care workforce issues between 1973 and 1990; and William Schwartz, a physician at Tufts New England Medical Center, who conducted research on economics and health care, especially on rationing health care from 1976 to 1989.[6] The payoff from these grants was extremely high, providing insights into the health care system and ideas for potential programming. Important as these grants were, they constituted about 0.3 percent of the Foundation's grantmaking from 1972 to 1990.

In 1972, the Foundation took its first step toward developing a corps of health services *researchers*—as contrasted with health services research—by taking over the Clinical Scholars Program from the Carnegie Corporation and the Commonwealth Fund. This program strengthened the field by training a group of physicians as researchers and later by providing a model for training scholars from other fields.

In December of 1976, Linda Aiken, at the time the Foundation's director of research and later a vice president; David Rogers, its president; and Robert Blendon, its vice president, reported to the Foundation's board that the research grantmaking

> has been aimed quite directly at improving the staff's ability to develop good programs in our fields of interest and evaluation of these efforts. Added to this has been a strong targeted program to develop knowledge about issues of direct concern to us that can be shared with the professional and broader public groups. Thus it is not surprising that over 70 percent of our research grants have been directed at studies of ways to improve areas such as rural care, child health, community hospital outpatient care, emergency services, and general access to physician care, etc.

Supporting Health Services Research

In more than three decades, the Foundation has appropriated over $1.3 billion for research, most of which has been health services research. In 2006, the Foundation appropriated about $87 million for research. However, the Foundation's spending on health services research pales in comparison with that of the federal government. It is estimated that the Agency for Healthcare Research and Quality budgeted $135 million in 2006 for research grants and the Medical Expenditure Panel Survey, the National Institutes of Health budgeted about $938 million for health services research, and the Centers for Medicare & Medicaid Services allocated $1 million for investigator-initiated research.[7]

A few selected projects exemplify the Foundation's research activities. These projects are mainly practical ones that have helped the Foundation answer two questions in its priority areas:

- *What is the nature of the problem?* The access-to-care surveys, the Changes in Health Care Financing and Organization (HCFO) initiative, and Health Tracking are examples of projects that addressed this question. This research enabled the Foundation and the broader health policy community to gain a better understanding of costs, quality, and access to medical care.
- *What solutions work to solve a particular problem?* In addition to studying problems, HCFO evaluates specific solutions. The Cash & Counseling program and SUPPORT (the Study to Understand Prognoses and Preferences for Outcomes and Risks of Treatment) are examples of research-driven demonstration projects that tried to solve specific problems.

Access to Care

In its early years, the Foundation was concerned with access to health care, especially primary care. In 1973, it funded the first of four access-to-care surveys.[8] That survey, conducted by Ronald Andersen and Lu Ann Aday of the University of Chicago, found that 78 percent of Americans had a principal physician whom they could identify by name. About 12 percent had a need for care but did not have a regular source of care. At least 3 percent did not have any source of care. Seven percent did not need care. Poor children and poor elders had worse access to care than other Americans.[9]

As part of its focus on access, the Foundation also funded the University of Southern California professor of medicine Robert Mendenhall and his colleagues to survey physicians about how much time they spent on primary care services. Although the study showed that an overwhelming amount of primary care was provided by generalist physicians, one in five patients received primary care from a specialist. As a result, the Foundation learned that, because of the contribution of specialists, the shortage of primary care was not as great as had previously been thought.

These surveys—the first national surveys to concentrate on access to care—provided valuable information that guided the Foundation's programming. They developed important measures of access to care that are still used today, and they later informed the work of the Center for Studying Health System Change.[10]

Health Care Financing and Organization

The first large initiative supporting health services research was the Program for Demonstration and Research on Health Care Costs, which began in 1982.[11] Originally a small grant program run internally by Foundation staff members, it was later transformed into a larger initiative managed by a national program office at the Alpha Center, a health research and policy organization in Washington, D.C. Over its lifetime (the last grant ended in 1992), it awarded forty-four grants for more than $10 million. Although the projects under this program ranged widely, the program created a body of work that focused on prospective payment, capitation, and case management.

Nevertheless, the Program for Demonstration and Research on Health Care Costs failed to receive enough high-quality proposals. Foundation staff members felt that this was due to the program's narrow focus on cost savings. Building on the experience of that program, in 1988 the Foundation authorized the Changes in Health Care Financing and Organization (HCFO) program, which had a broader focus of encouraging demonstrations, research, and evaluations on health care financing, organization, and impact. Originally authorized at a $12 million level for three years, HCFO has been extended five times, with a total funding of $76 million. It has funded more than 265 projects on how financing has affected cost, access, organization, and quality. These projects have investigated various aspects of health insurance, consumer behavior, health care markets, managed care, Medicaid, Medicare, organization and delivery of care, provider payment, and regulation of health care. The Alpha Center served as the National Program Office through 2000, when it merged with the Association for Health Services Research to become AcademyHealth, which continues to manage the program.

Among the areas that HCFO has funded is a large body of work on risk adjustment. Because policymakers were worried that some health plans would enroll primarily healthy patients, researchers were asked to develop compensatory mechanisms, called risk adjustment, so that insurers serving unhealthier patients and running the risk of higher costs would be compensated appropriately for taking those risks. Under HCFO grants, risk-adjustment methods were developed that were used by the Health Insurance Plan of California and the Pacific Business Group on Health. HCFO also funded evaluations of high-risk pools—a mechanism used by some states to insure people in poor health who otherwise would not be able to obtain health insurance. The evaluations showed that high-risk pools helped a small number of middle- and high-income individuals acquire insurance coverage but did not help low-income individuals.

In its early and middle years, HCFO used meetings and conferences extensively as a way to provide decision makers with timely information relevant to policymaking. Between 1994 and 2006, for example, it organized at least half a dozen meetings on risk adjustment. In addition, HCFO used newsletters, briefs, and special papers, as well as peer-reviewed journal articles, to disseminate findings to policymakers. A summary of the first risk-adjustment meeting, held in 1994, and some of the meeting papers were published in the spring 1995 issue of *Inquiry.* This was followed by a HCFO special report in 1997, another issue of *Inquiry* in the summer of 1998, and a HCFO issue brief on risk adjustment in 2005.

In a 1996 evaluation, Kathryn Langwell, an economist at the Barents Group, and James Morone, a professor at Brown University, concluded,

"HCFO represents a stable source of funding for health financing and organizational research which, given the federal budget deficit and current uncertainties, is a very important 'niche' from the perspective of the research community."[12] Still, Langwell and Morone concluded that HCFO had a mixed record on influencing policymaking. According to them, HCFO researchers lacked bridges to the policy community. By contrast, a later evaluation of HCFO by Jack Hoadley and Michael Gluck of Georgetown University found that policymakers felt that the work funded through HCFO was important to policy making. They wrote, for example, that "[Harvard economist Katherine] Swartz's project on the dynamics of spells without health insurance is an example of a project that affected analysts' understanding of what it means to be uninsured."

Health Tracking

In 1994, the Foundation established the Health Tracking initiative to monitor the impact of changes in the health care system and how they affect Americans' health. The Foundation has authorized more than $136 million for this program. As the main engine of the Health Tracking initiative, the Center for Studying Health System Change conducts in-depth quantitative and qualitative research on twelve communities, as well as studies on a wide variety of health financing and organization issues.

In addition to the research conducted by the Center, the RAND Corporation conducted studies on mental health and addiction, medical group practices, employer-based health insurance, and quality of care. A widely reported study by researcher Elizabeth McGlynn and her colleagues at RAND, for example, showed that Americans received only about 55 percent of the care recommended for chronic conditions.[13]

The Center's research has been published in more than 170 peer-reviewed articles, and it posts numerous reports and issues briefs on its Web site. Serving as a think tank on health care issues, the Center has conducted briefings for the staffs of the Department of Health and Human Services, the Treasury Department, the Office of Management and Budget, and the Joint Committee on Taxation, and its staff members have testified before congressional committees.

In its early days, the Center had not mastered the art of distilling its reports into a form useful to policymakers; consequently, it did not fulfill its potential as a source of policy-relevant information. It appears to have overcome that problem and is widely considered to be a very influential organization in Washington health policy circles.[14] AcademyHealth presented the 2006 Health Services Research Impact Award to the Center for its work on specialty hospitals. This work stimulated Congress to place a moratorium on new specialty hospitals participating in Medicare until after the Centers for Medicare & Medicaid Services and the Medicare Payment Advisory Commission conducted studies on payment and related issues.[15]

Cash & Counseling

A research-driven demonstration project, Cash & Counseling is a program that provides a budget for homebound elders and disabled adults with chronic conditions to buy the home-health services they need. With support from the Foundation and the federal government, experimental Cash & Counseling programs were developed in three states that enabled homebound Medicaid recipients to pay people of their own choosing (such as a relative) instead of an agency for home health services. An evaluation conducted by Randall Brown and his colleagues at Mathematica Policy Research found that Cash & Counseling reduced unmet needs of consumers and improved the quality of life for both the consumers and the caregivers. Costs were somewhat higher than for traditional home health care, but these were partially offset by reductions in nursing home care and could be controlled in a well-designed program.[16] Today, twelve states are replicating the programs of the original states with Medicaid waivers, and a provision of the Deficit Reduction Act of 2005 allows all states to adopt the approach without a waiver starting in 2007.

SUPPORT

The Study to Understand Prognoses and Preferences for Outcomes and Risks of Treatments (SUPPORT) used specially trained nurses to counsel terminally ill hospitalized patients and their families in an attempt to improve decision making toward the end of life. This was a large demonstration-research project whose results were carefully monitored. Contrary to expectations, the study revealed that the intervention did not improve decision making about the care that dying patients should or should not receive and that the wishes of patients and their families were routinely ignored.[17] After receiving the negative results from SUPPORT, the Foundation recognized that it had an opportunity to improve the care given to terminally ill patients and it developed a variety of programs with that objective.[18]

Developing a Corps of Health Services Researchers

As early as January of 1973, the Foundation's board recognized that supporting research itself was not enough and that there was a need to train a new generation of personnel to conduct research. At the time, most researchers were trained to do basic research that was published in scholarly journals and addressed to other university-based researchers. From the Foundation's perspective, the greatest need was to train individuals who would be interested in conducting applied research or policy analysis and communicating the results of that research to decision makers.

Training Physicians, Dentists, and Nurses in the Social Sciences

To create a new generation of physician-scholars and leaders, in 1972 the Foundation committed itself to funding the Robert Wood Johnson Clinical Scholars Program, which the Carnegie Corporation and the Commonwealth Fund had started in 1969 as a three-year pilot program. Through this program, these physician-scholars would learn the tools that are necessary to conduct health services and health policy research. The program would expand their knowledge to include nonclinical areas of health, such as the economics and financing of health care. This early strategy to train only physicians in health services research assumed that physicians would dominate the field—an assumption that was not borne out. Nevertheless, the Clinical Scholars program has become a signature program of the Foundation, and its basic design was copied in several of the training programs that the Foundation developed later.[19]

Many Clinical Scholars have become leaders in the field of health services research and in health policy. In a 1992 evaluation of the program, two distinguished health policy experts, John Rowe and Rashi Fein, pronounced it a "tremendous success" and noted that it had legitimized health services research. Later, Jonathan Showstack, a health services research expert, and his colleagues at the University of California, San Francisco also found that the Clinical Scholars program had legitimized health services research in medicine and produced leading researchers in the field.[20] Today, there are more than a thousand former Clinical Scholars, and many have become leading health services researchers, such as Robert Brook of Rand Health, Mark Chassin of the Mount Sinai School of Medicine, and the late John Eisenberg of the Agency for Healthcare Research and Quality. Three others—Risa Lavizzo-Mourey of the Robert Wood Johnson Foundation, Mark Smith of the California HealthCare Foundation, and Robert Ross of the California Endowment—are presidents of organizations that fund health services research.

Established in 1982, the Dental Services Research Scholars and the Clinical Nurse Scholars programs were designed along the lines of the Clinical Scholars program. The goal of the Dental Services Research Scholars program was to develop leaders of dental school faculties; to this end, the program focused on the study of health services organization, economics and finance, epidemiology, and policy analysis. Dental Research Scholars were expected to master methodological skills, gain knowledge in a chosen area of concentration, and complete a publishable research product in a two-year fellowship program. Fundamentally, the Dental Services Research Scholars were being trained to become health services researchers with a specialty in dental services.

By the end of the program, in 1990, two sites at the dental schools of Harvard University and the University of California, Los Angeles, had thirty graduates. The Foundation closed this program because of its success (training three times as many dental health services researchers as there had been ten years before) at a time when demand was decreasing. Dental school enrollment was dropping and, indeed, at the time dental schools were closing.

The Clinical Nurse Scholars Program was designed to redirect the research of nursing faculty members to clinical problems that would improve the outcome of clinical care. This was a two-year program at three sites—the University of Pennsylvania; the University of California, San Francisco; and the University of Rochester. It was first a mid-career program and then became a postdoctoral program.[21] This program had sixty-two graduates when it closed in 1991. The Clinical Nurse Scholars program did not have a significant impact on health services research, but its graduates were very successful in competing for National Institutes of Health funding. The research topics chosen by the Clinical Nurse Scholars focused more on clinical areas than on health services.

In 1993, as part of its efforts to make primary care more attractive, the Robert Wood Johnson Foundation authorized the Generalist Physician Faculty Scholars Program to enhance the career development of generalist junior faculty physicians. For the purpose of this program the term *generalist physicians* included family physicians, general internists, and general pediatricians. Each medical school could nominate one person a year for the program, which provided four-year awards that were meant to increase the research skills of the participating faculty. Scholars received $60,000 a year to buy themselves out of clinical duties and teaching responsibilities, to conduct research, and to receive mentoring by a member of the National Advisory Committee.

By the time the program closes, in 2008, it will have awarded 175 fellowships, with about a third of those going to former Clinical Scholars. Although there was no programmatic reason (albeit there might be a career reason), most of the research conducted by Generalist Physician Faculty Scholars was on clinical rather than health services research topics. Nonetheless, some former Generalist Physician Faculty Scholars, such as Kevin Grumbach of the University of California, San Francisco, have become leaders in health services research.

Developing Social Science Researchers

The first attempt to train social science faculty members in health services research was the Program for Faculty Fellowships in Health Care Finance, a small program with only one location, the Johns Hopkins University.

In its first year, the program included background orientation on health care finance followed by internships and, in its second year, a small research grant for each fellow. The program ran from 1984 to 1994, training sixty fellows, but it was judged to be unsuccessful and was ended.[22] Although the program did not have a big impact on health services research, some of the fellows have continued to influence the field—for example, Robert Ohsfeldt at Texas A&M Health Sciences Center, whose recent book, *The Business of Health,* argues for strengthening competitive forces in the U.S. health care market;[23] Mark Hall of Wake Forest University School of Law, an expert in health care law; and Kyle Grazier of the University of Michigan School of Public Health, the editor of the *Journal of Healthcare Management.*

The Robert Wood Johnson Scholars in Health Policy Research Program is a two-year fellowship program designed to attract top economists, political scientists, and sociologists to the fields of health policy and health services research. It was authorized in 1991, and the first cohort entered the program in 1994. There are three sites; they provide an introduction to health policy and services research, mentoring by senior faculty, and resources for research projects. Up to twelve scholars enter the program each year, and 153 Scholars had participated in this program as of 2006.

In an early evaluation, Stephen Shortell, currently the dean of the school of public health at the University of California, Berkeley, and Burton Weisbrod, a professor of economics at Northwestern University, judged it to be "on a productive path." In a later evaluation, John Palmer, who is currently the dean emeritus of Syracuse University's Maxwell School, and his colleagues concluded that "our overall assessment of this program is quite high."

Some of the scholars—such as Daniel Carpenter, a professor of government at Harvard University—have introduced health topics in arts and sciences departments; others, such as Paula Lantz, who chairs the department of health policy and management at the University of Michigan's School of Public Health, are mainstream health services researchers. John Cawley, an associate professor of policy analysis and management at Cornell University, conducts research on the economics of obesity. In 2005, he received the John D. Thompson Prize for Young Investigators in Health Services Research.

In 2001, the Foundation's board of trustees authorized the Robert Wood Johnson Health and Society Scholars Program to encourage the development of scholars and researchers in the field of population health. This is an interdisciplinary training program involving the social, behavioral, and health sciences. The model is similar to the one used in the Clinical Scholars and the Scholars in Health Policy Research programs. It provides a two-year fellowship with an introduction to the field of population health, along with research opportunities for up to eighteen scholars a year at six universities. As of 2006, eighty scholars had entered the program.

Investigator Awards in Health Policy Research

The Investigator Awards in Health Policy Research program was authorized in 1991 to replace the "great men awards."[24] As a research program, it funds about ten projects a year that conduct innovative research like that done under the great men awards. As a human capital program, it tries to keep senior scholars in the field and to attract new talent to it. The program has funded over 140 individual Investigators who have produced more than fifty books and over four hundred articles.

Investigators' publications are widely cited and influential. For example, Dalton Conley was the first sociologist and the second social scientist to win the National Science Foundation's Alan T. Waterman Award, recognizing a young researcher in science or engineering. The NSF cited his Investigator work that resulted in *The Pecking Order*[25] and *The Starting Gate*,[26] two books showing how inequalities in families develop.

Investigator Awards' research projects have focused on public health problems, quality of care, financing issues, and health disparities, among other topics. Several Investigators have created a body of work on disparities, generally showing that when it comes to health, socioeconomic status is an important factor in determining health.

Building the Field

Although the Robert Wood Johnson Foundation has played an important role in funding health services research in its interest areas and in training scholars in health services research, its support for the field of health services research has been inconsistent. For much of its history, the Foundation has not seen building and supporting the field as crucial to achieving its programmatic goals.

Still, Foundation support for health services research, though sporadic until recently, has been crucial at times. By early 1983, the federal government had dramatically reduced its support for health services research. The budget for the National Center for Health Services Research dropped from $56 million in 1972 to $10 million in 1982. At that time, the staff felt that the Foundation had a major stake in the success of the field of health services research and that many federal policymakers did not understand the value of health services research. In response to this situation, in 1982 the Foundation made a small grant to the Foundation for Health Services Research—the charitable arm of the Association for Health Services Research—to build and support the field. The main purpose of the grant was to improve the relationship between researchers and the users of research.

After that project, there was no further Foundation funding of this kind in the 1980s and early 1990s. With the initiation of the Investigator Awards and the Scholars in Health Policy Research programs in the 1990s, the Foundation recognized the need to build capacity within the field of health policy research. In 1999, the Foundation awarded the first of two small grants to AcademyHealth to develop a campaign to increase the understanding of health services research. Under this campaign, called *Connecting the Dots,* AcademyHealth created a logo, produced flyers, developed stories about how health services research had influenced policy and practice, and identified champions of health services research. With little external financial support for this campaign, the small grant from the Foundation was crucial for its implementation. Although the impact of this meagerly funded campaign is not known, for the first time it provided communications and outreach to support the field.

Beginning in 2004, the Foundation decided to consolidate its support for all activities of AcademyHealth—including its dues, support for the National Health Policy Conference, scholarships for students at the research meeting, and efforts of the organization to be a force in the transmission of research to the policy community. Later, this consolidated grant was expanded to allow AcademyHealth to convene key sponsors of research, including leaders from federal agencies and foundations; to address future challenges to the field; and to develop a strategic plan for health services research.

Supporting Professional Journals

A lack of consistent commitment, with a few brief interventions at crucial points, also characterizes the Foundation's history of support for health services research journals. The most notable support has been for *Health Affairs,* a health policy journal that is a broker of information between researchers and policymakers, but that has been more recent. *Health Affairs* began in 1981 as a dissemination vehicle for the Center for Health Information, Research and Analysis (which became the Center for Health Affairs in 1984) at Project Hope. In 1982, the Foundation gave a grant for the development of this center, which included a small amount to support *Health Affairs.* Although the center no longer exists, *Health Affairs* is a thriving enterprise.

From then until early 2000, the Foundation's support for *Health Affairs* was directed toward specific projects. Since 1989, the Robert Wood Johnson Foundation, along with other foundations, has consistently supported the GrantWatch section of *Health Affairs.* From 1993 to 1996, the Foundation supported the coverage of intergovernmental policy issues in *Health Affairs.* With Foundation support, *Health Affairs* published supplemental issues on managed competition, the Clinton Administration's health care proposal, competition in managed care, the reform of medical education, and the employer-based health system. After the development of the Health Tracking project, based at the Center for Studying Health System Change, the Foundation looked for outlets for the Center's work. To address that need, the Foundation funded the Health Tracking section in every issue of *Health Affairs.*

Until 1995, the Foundation provided support for *Health Affairs* on a case-by-case, project-specific basis. Then, as a way to provide stable funding for the journal, the Foundation made a core-support grant to *Health Affairs,* and it has continued that practice through the present.

The Foundation has also supported market research for *Health Affairs* on several occasions. In 1995, the Foundation funded focus groups of subscribers and the collection of data on readership. Under this grant, demographic information about subscribers and their interests, as well as nonsubscribers' perceptions of the journal, was collected. Readers saw *Health Affairs* as a valuable resource but indicated that it needed a more reader-friendly format. More recently, the Foundation financed a study of the journal's business practices.

Health Affairs has become an effective vehicle to transmit knowledge from researchers to policymakers. It publishes more than 250 articles a year, including articles in a Web-exclusive version, and convenes press and policy briefings. It has a subscriber base of eleven thousand, more than any other health services research journal.

Health Affairs is influential in policymaking. From January to late November of 2006 it was cited in congressional testimony at about the same level as the *New England Journal of Medicine* and the *Journal of the American Medical Association.* Twenty-seven *Health Affairs* articles were cited in congressional testimony, compared with the next closest health services research journal, *Health Services Research,* which had one citation during the time period. Fifty-five percent of congressional staff members on health committees read *Health Affairs,* whereas only 17 percent read the *Journal of the American Medical Association* and 10 percent read the *New England Journal of Medicine.*

Foundation support for other journals—such as *Health Services Research, Inquiry,* and the *Journal of Health Politics, Policy and Law*—has been more limited and sporadic. For example, over nearly three decades, the Foundation has funded six special issues of the *Journal of Health Politics, Policy and Law.* It financed three special issues of *Health Services Research* dedicated to the memory of Alice Hersh, the first executive director of the Association for Health Services Research. Later, the Foundation, jointly with the Agency for Healthcare Research and Quality's predecessor agency, funded a special issue of *Health Services Research* on the use of qualitative research in health services research. That issue has had an impact in setting the methodological standards for qualitative health services research as well as gaining legitimacy for that type of research.

Conclusion

The Foundation's impact on the development of health services *researchers* has been deliberate and long-term. Many of the field's leaders are alumni of the Foundation's human capital programs. These programs have given individuals methodological training and education in substantive areas that they would not have received otherwise. The Foundation's programs have created career paths for the next generation of health services researchers and have provided legitimacy for health services research, especially in medicine. Some programs are even trying to develop research and researchers in new fields, such as population health.

The Foundation's influence on health services *research* has also been profound. One indicator of the Foundation's impact on health services research comes from the National Library of Medicine's Health Services Research Projects in Progress, which indicates that the Robert Wood Johnson Foundation has funded 1,404 research projects that are in progress; the next closest funder is the Agency for Healthcare Research and Quality, with 1,260. In contrast, the Commonwealth Fund has 257; the California HealthCare Foundation, 97; the Kellogg Foundation, 8; the Pew Charitable Trusts, 7; and the Kaiser Family Foundation and the California Endowment, 1 each.[27]

Research can influence the way decision makers see the problem, as shown by the work of Katherine Swartz on the way people go on and off of health insurance, Robert Mendenhall and his colleagues' work on primary care, or Elizabeth McGlynn's work on quality of care. It can influence policy decisions, as demonstrated by Paul Ginsburg and his colleagues at the Center for Studying Health System Change in their research on specialty hospitals or that of Randall Brown and his colleagues on the impact of Cash & Counseling.

And it can influence practices of providers and health plans, as the risk adjustment work done by many grantees under HCFO illustrates. But the route from developing knowledge to having impact is generally long and tortuous. Ideas are created, but entrepreneurs need to connect the ideas with those in a position to put them to use in policies.[28]

Although the Foundation's influence on the *field* of health services research has also been great, it has come about in an incidental manner. For many years, the Foundation did not intend to support the development of a field; it financed health services research and researchers. Though it may be in the Foundation's self-interest to promote health services research as a field, its reluctance to provide core support until recently has restrained its influence. However, the Foundation's consolidation, or core support, grants to the Association for Health Services Research, AcademyHealth, and *Health Affairs* have supported the development of the field. On the whole, the Robert Wood Johnson Foundation's support for the field of health services research has been sporadic but crucial.

Notes

1. Ginzberg, E. "Health Services Research and Health Policy." *Health Services Research.* Cambridge, Mass.: Harvard University Press, 1991, 2.
2. Brown, L. D. "Knowledge and Power: Health Services Research as a Political Resource." *Health Services Research.* Cambridge, Mass.: Harvard University Press, 1991, 35–36.
3. Institute of Medicine. *Health Services Research: Work Force and Educational Issues.* Washington, D.C.: National Academy Press, 1995, 3.
4. The Robert Wood Johnson Foundation. *The Robert Wood Johnson Foundation Annual Report,* 1973, 24. (http://www.rwjf.org/files/publications/annual/AnnualReport1973.pdf?gsa=1)
5. Later the Foundation also funded Georgetown University to develop a policy center.
6. Colby, D. C. "Building Health Policy Research Capacity in the Social Sciences." *To Improve Health and Health Care, Vol. VI: The Robert Wood Johnson Foundation.* San Francisco: Jossey-Bass, 2003, 183–187.
7. Coalition for Health Services Research. Federal Funding for Health Services Research. December 2006, p. 1.
8. Anderson and Aday conducted the first two surveys. The third survey was conducted by Howard Freeman at the University of California, Los Angeles. The fourth was conducted by Marc Berk of Project Hope.
9. The Robert Wood Johnson Foundation. *The Robert Wood Johnson Foundation Annual Report,* 1979, 9–10. (http://www.rwjf.org/files/publications/annual/AnnualReport1979.pdf?gsa=1)

10. For a review of these surveys, see Berk, M. L. and Schur, C. L., "A Review of the National Access-to-Care Surveys." *To Improve Health and Health Care 1997: The Robert Wood Johnson Foundation Anthology.* San Francisco: Jossey-Bass, 1997, 53–77.
11. There were earlier national research programs, but they were more focused on clinical matters. For example, the Medical Practice Research and Demonstration program supported projects studying falls among the elderly and the use of relaxation techniques to reduce the frequency and severity of asthma attacks.
12. Barents Group. Evaluation of the Robert Wood Johnson's Health Care Financing and Organization Initiative (HCFO). Washington, D.C., 1996, 14.
13. McGlynn, E. A., and others. "The Quality of Health Care Delivered to Adults in the United States." *New England Journal of Medicine,* 2003, *348*(26): 2635–2645.
14. Newbergh, C., "The Health Tracking Initiative." *To Improve Health and Health Care, Vol. VI: The Robert Wood Johnson Foundation Anthology.* San Francisco: Jossey-Bass, 2003, 29–49.
15. AcademyHealth, "Specialty Hospitals: 2006 HSR Impact Awardee."
16. Benjamin, A. E., and Fennel, M. L. "Putting Consumers First in Long-Term Care: Findings fron the Cash & Counseling Demonstrations and Evaluation." *Health Service Research,* 2007, *42*(1), Part II.
17. Lynn, J. "Unexpected Returns: Insights from SUPPORT." *To Improve Health and Health Care 1997: The Robert Wood Johnson Foundation Anthology.* San Francisco: Jossey-Bass, 1997, 161–186.
18. Bronner, E, "The Foundation's End-of-Life Programs: Changing the American Way of Death." *To Improve Health and Health Care, Vol. VI: The Robert Wood Johnson Foundation Anthology.* San Francisco: Jossey-Bass, 2003, 81–98.
19. Showstack, J., Rothman, A. A., Leviton, L. G., and Sandy, L. G. "The Robert Wood Johnson Clinical Scholars Program." *To Improve Health and Health Care, Vol. VII: The Robert Wood Johnson Foundation Anthology.* San Francisco: Jossey-Bass, 2004, 105–123.
20. Ibid, 112–113.
21. Isaacs, S. L., Sandy, L. G., and Schroeder, S. A. "Improving the Health Care Workforce." *To Improve Health and Health Care 1997: The Robert Wood Johnson Foundation Anthology.* San Francisco: Jossey-Bass, 1997, 31–33.
22. Colby, D. C. "Building Health Policy Research Capacity in the Social Sciences." *To Improve Health and Health Care, Vol. VI: The Robert Wood Johnson Foundation Anthology.* San Francisco: Jossey-Bass, 2003, 187–189.
23. Ohlsfeldt, R. L., and Schneider, J. E. *The Business of Health: The Role of Competition, Markets, and Regulation.* Washington, D.C.: AEI Press, 2006.
24. For more information on the Investigator Awards in Health Policy Research program, see Colby, D. C. "Building Health Policy Research Capacity in the Social Sciences." *To Improve Health and Health Care, Vol. VI: The Robert Wood Johnson Foundation Anthology.* San Francisco: Jossey-Bass, 2003.

25. Conley, D. *The Pecking Order: A Bold New Look at How Family and Society Determine Who We Become.* New York: Random House, 2005.
26. Conley, D., Strully, K. W., and Bennett, N. G. *The Starting Gate: Birth Weight and Life Chances.* Berkeley, Calif.: University of California Press, 2003.
27. National Library of Medicine. National Information Center on Health Services Research and Health Care Technology (NICHSR). (http://www.nlm.nih.gov/hsrproj/). March 3, 2007.
28. For discussions of this, see the following: Cohen, M. D., March, J. G, and Olson, J. P. "The Garbage Can Model of Organizational Choice." *Administrative Science Quarterly, 17,* 1–25; Kingdon, J. *Agendas, Alternatives, and Public Policies.* Boston: Little, Brown, 1984; and Brown, L. D. "Knowledge and Power: Health Services Research as a Political Resource." *Health Services Research.* Cambridge, Mass.: Harvard University Press, 1991, 20–45.

CHAPTER 3

Reducing Teenage Pregnancy

Will Bunch

Editors' Introduction

Teenage pregnancy raises important social, economic, moral, and family concerns. Any foundation endeavoring to address adolescent pregnancy must recognize the potentially explosive nature of the issue and, if it wishes to avoid being caught in an explosion, proceed with delicacy. In this chapter, Will Bunch, a Pulitzer Prize–winning journalist with the *Philadelphia Daily News,* traces the evolution of the Robert Wood Johnson Foundation's efforts over a twenty-year period to address this potentially controversial issue.

Although it has never been one of its explicit priorities, the Foundation has allocated more than $179 million to reducing teenage pregnancy. Its initial efforts—supporting school-based health centers that, among other things, referred high school students to contraceptive counseling and services—generated considerable controversy when they were introduced in the 1980s. Although the Foundation has continued to support school-based health centers and has also funded an abstinence-only program, in the 1990s it settled on an approach that tended to tamp down potential controversy: it supported the National Campaign to Prevent Teen Pregnancy, which involves people from all parts of the political spectrum, uses the latest scientific information in presenting the issues, recommends multiple approaches to reducing teen pregnancy, and frames the debate in terms of the social and economic costs of teen pregnancy.

In addition to providing insights about reducing teenage pregnancy, this chapter also illustrates how the Foundation has approached a potentially controversial area that it considers important. Two other examples of the Foundation entering a controversial area come to mind. One is coverage of the uninsured: the Foundation, after having been accused of promoting the Clinton health care plan in the 1990s, adopted a less controversial approach based on information campaigns supporting children's health insurance and convening a broad range of organizations with markedly different political perspectives to develop a consensus position on health insurance coverage. The other area is tobacco control. The Foundation directly challenged the tobacco industry at a time when it was far less unpopular than it is today. To minimize controversy, however, the Foundation set its work within the context of protecting children and employed a coalition-building approach that encompassed a wide range of organizations in the public health and tobacco-control communities.

At the Pathways/Senderos Center in the timeworn downtown of New Britain, Connecticut, the afternoon begins with hugs—and with heaping bowls of cereal. At roughly 2:30 every afternoon, high school students begin bounding up the rear steps to the program's second-floor location—an odd jumble of offices, stocked food pantries, busy computer terminals, and rec-room-style couches. The hugs, or *abrazos,* are a custom in this heavily Latino, poverty-plagued neighborhood, while the cereal is much-needed nutrition. By 3:30, middle school students begin trickling in, until the big room fills with nearly fifty kids—roughly half boys and half girls, some quietly doing homework at a corner table, while two boys practice a dance routine in front of several giggling pals.

An unknowing visitor could spend an entire afternoon here without realizing the true purpose of the Pathway/Senderos Center. Pathways/Senderos is one of dozens of local programs across the country that have benefited from a two-way relationship with the National Campaign to Prevent Teen Pregnancy—a relationship that involves an ongoing exchange of ideas and best practices, although not dollars. It is a program to prevent teenage pregnancy, and despite its location in an impoverished stretch of a fading New England factory town, the fact that it is arguably one of the most successful in the country is a gratifying testament to the effectiveness of the program. Since the Connecticut program was launched in 1993, only three of roughly two hundred girls and boys who have cycled through the multiyear, intensive after-school program have either become pregnant or fathered a child—even though a majority of the students are products of teen parents themselves.

The novel approach of the Connecticut program—focusing on staying in school over traditional sex education—closely follows the model promoted by the sweeping, decade-old program it maintains close ties to: the National Campaign to Prevent Teen Pregnancy. Since the Washington-based National Campaign was launched in February 1996 as a nonprofit, nonpartisan group arising from an initiative by President Bill Clinton, the Robert Wood Johnson Foundation has been one of its major patrons. Not only did the Foundation provide more than one-quarter of the roughly $20 million spent by the National Campaign in its first decade, but the

Campaign has received the lion's share of the Foundation's funding of programs to prevent teen pregnancy.

Although reducing teen pregnancy has never been an explicit priority of the Foundation, it is an area in which its investment has coincided with remarkable progress, as both statistics and exhaustive study have documented. When the Campaign was launched, eleven years ago, the rate of unmarried teen births was near its peak after rising sharply in the 1980s, and it was much higher in the United States than in any other industrialized country. Nevertheless, the Campaign set an ambitious goal of reducing teen pregnancy rates by one-third by 2005—a target that, according to the latest data, appears to have been reached.

The Campaign does not and cannot take all—or even most—of the credit for that drop, apparently the result of a combination of changing social attitudes and sexual practices and of successful local efforts like the one in New Britain. But leading authorities in the field credit the Campaign with helping to change the nature of the debate about teen pregnancy, which in the 1980s and into the middle 1990s had become bogged down in America's socially charged culture wars over sex, abstinence, contraception for teenagers, and abortion.

Sharon Camp, the president of the Guttmacher Institute, a research and public policy organization that focuses on sexual and reproductive health, said that the Campaign, with its approach of incorporating both abstinence education and contraception, enabled state and local officials to first talk about teen pregnancy and then carry out new programs. She said the Campaign's effective politicking helped existing groups such as Planned Parenthood since the improved climate allowed lawmakers in some states to increase teenagers' access to confidential counseling and services. "They [the Campaign] provided permission, in a sense," Camp said.

Allan Rosenfield, the dean of the Mailman School of Public Health at Columbia University, largely agreed with Camp's analysis. He said he believes that the Campaign, with its sweeping efforts from the Internet to story placement on daytime television, raised awareness of the issue and helped bring more teens into established programs such as Planned Parenthood. That is critical, he explained, because the heightened awareness comes at a time when some schools are eliminating traditional sex education, while larger numbers of traditional gynecologists are hesitant to provide contraception without parental consent. Rosenfield noted that it's hard to quantify the work of any one group, but "a lot of groups have used the materials that the Campaign provided, and that has helped them work together."

Indeed, the relationship that the Campaign has forged with local groups—from Planned Parenthood chapters to community-based efforts like Pathways/Senderos—is a complicated one, in which money does not change hands, as it might with more traditional public health networks. Instead, the Campaign sees its role as setting the broad strategy, in areas from research to public awareness. The local groups are the tacticians on the front line. The Campaign sometimes learns about best practices from outlets like Pathways/Senderos, and it recycles those techniques to other agencies.

From its very beginning, the Campaign placed strong emphasis on teenage pregnancy as a socioeconomic problem that affected the broader society. It saw its role as bridging the gap between abstinence-only programs and those that endorsed sex counseling and contraception—promoting whatever practices were effective, encouraging scientific research, and sharing knowledge and best practices with community groups. The Campaign was born of the same instincts to seek a middle ground on a thorny political issue that led to national welfare reform in the mid-to-late 1990s, and officials both with the Campaign and at the Foundation believe its greatest contribution may have been making the American debate about teen pregnancy less about the divisive issue of sex education and contraception and more about how reducing teen births would decrease poverty and related social ills.

At the Pathway/Senderos program in New Britain, that philosophy comes alive. Its motto, displayed prominently on the wall and on T-shirts, is "Diplomas Before Diapers." In fact, the students there spend two hours a week in a "Job Club," earning $2 an hour to develop basic work skills, and only one hour a week in a sex education and family life class. Much of the rest of the week is spent on academics and promoting the idea that college is the only sure path to success in this city of seventy-one thousand where decent-paying factory jobs have vanished and the largest private employers are retailers and fast-food outlets such as Wal-Mart, McDonald's, and Dunkin' Donuts.

In interviews with half a dozen of the kids taking part in Pathways/Senderos, most talk with enthusiasm about job goals after high school, such as culinary arts or veterinary medicine—and most have come to view pregnancy and raising a child through that prism of career choices. Typical is seventeen-year-old Reggie Roberts, a senior at New Britain High School, who sees no place for parenthood as he prepares college applications with an eye toward child psychology. He said he had peers who thought they could stay in school and raise a child, "but if you actually have a baby it's not going to be like that."

Like the first teen pregnancy prevention programs, which were born in the 1970s, the Pathways/Senderos program does not shy away from the subject of contraception for those teens who are sexually active. The program distributes condoms to students who ask for them and encourages any teenager having sex to use two forms of birth control; during the year there will be a field trip to a family planning clinic and to New Britain's main hospital. Yet one reason that the program is effective may be that sex is such a small part of the curriculum. "I never mention sex," executive director RoseAnne Bilodeau says as she touts the program's highlights.

Local programs like hers are not directly funded by the National Campaign to Prevent Teen Pregnancy, but there is a close line of communication: the Campaign often asks Bilodeau to speak at events, and her program is held up as a model to other community groups as an example of an approach that works.

Interestingly, the strategies of the 1990s and 2000s were shaped directly by the controversies of the 1980s, when the Foundation waded right into the middle of the acrimony and social warfare of that era by directly funding school-based clinics that, among other things, offered family-planning counseling and referrals for contraception—which drew fire from conservatives. The Campaign would prove to be a much less contentious approach.

Schools and Teenage Pregnancy

The issue of teen pregnancy and its relationship to broader social issues in America is a complex one. In fact, in the United States the rates of young women under the age of twenty becoming pregnant and giving birth reached their peak during the 1950s, coinciding with the baby boom that took place at the end of the Second World War. Many of these births were to teenagers who were already married, as a result of a social norm in which marriage and beginning a family at a very young age were far more common than they are today. Starting in the 1950s, there were diverging trends in America. Middle-class and upper-middle-class women were more likely to defer marriage and childbearing into their twenties and beyond, yet the rate of unmarried teen births rose, largely in poverty-stricken inner-city or rural communities.

In 1950, some 13 percent of American women aged nineteen and younger who gave birth were not married, but by 1988 that had climbed to 65 percent, and the raw number of babies born to this group soared from just under 60,000 to more than 300,000. The birth rate among American teens in the 1980s was much higher than that of other industrialized nations—more than twice the rate of England or Canada, and more than five times the rate of France.[1]

These new unmarried teen mothers typically raised their children in an environment in which fathers were absent and the expanding national welfare system was the main method of support. One study found that 77 percent of unmarried adolescent parents were welfare recipients within five years of giving birth.[2] In the 1980s, policymakers began to look at an "underclass" in American cities, with high rates of drug abuse and crime, and began to collect increasing evidence that high teen pregnancy rates encouraged this cycle of poverty.

During the same decade, the Foundation had begun an initiative to finance, in partnership with local foundations, community-run health centers in urban settings. The lessons from that first pilot project, called the Community Care Funding Partners Program, led the Foundation to finance a second program aimed at placing small health centers directly in schools. But in doing so the Foundation also entered the increasingly heated debate over teenage sex and pregnancy prevention programs.

The School-Based Adolescent Health Care Program was launched in 1986—the first step in the Foundation's twenty-plus-year commitment to school-based health care. It was intended as a broad-based initiative to address a range of health and behavioral problems that were afflicting inner city youth, including a lack of available mental health care, drug and alcohol abuse and addiction, and an estimated five million adolescents nationwide who had no health insurance. The following year, the Foundation awarded six-year grants to set up school-based clinics in twenty high schools in eighteen cities. Local health care providers were to run the clinics—typically staffed with a part-time physician, a nurse practitioner, a social worker, and a medical office assistant—in close coordination with school officials, a community advisory board, and local institutions that would ultimately take over the funding.[3]

The aspect of the plan that proved most controversial, however, was counseling adolescents on preventing unwanted pregnancy and sexually transmitted diseases, including advice on and referrals for contraception. These services were considered a requirement of the grant, but they would not be offered to students whose parents had not signed a consent form. That provision, as well as the role of community leaders in the advisory councils, was meant to head off controversy over the family-planning aspect of the program.

Julia Graham Lear, who served as codirector of the Foundation's School-Based Adolescent Health Care Program and who currently directs the Center for Health and Health Care in Schools at the George Washington University, said the plan that emerged in 1986 was something of a hybrid. Although she and a team of prominent Dallas-based pediatricians had lobbied for broadly based health centers in schools, Lear said that officials from the Center for Population Options, a nonprofit organization focused on reducing teenage pregnancy, wanted clinics in schools that would focus mainly on pregnancy prevention. At first, the Foundation's board of directors tabled the plan altogether, but then decided to proceed, as long as local community input was sought.

But in several key cities that wasn't enough to prevent the school-based clinics from becoming a political hot potato. Officials involved in the effort acknowledge that the Foundation was surprised by the strength of the opposition. That was especially true in Miami, where in 1987 the state's conservative governor, Republican Bob Martinez, used his powers to veto state aid for the health clinic that was planned for Northwestern High School there. He did so despite a poll of 619 parents that found two-thirds supported the clinic and despite backing for the new services from leaders in the local community. Given the strong community support, the Foundation was ultimately able to finance a health clinic there by channeling the money through a group that was not under state control.

There was controversy elsewhere as well, including Los Angeles, where the powerful archbishop of the Catholic Church, the future Cardinal Roger Mahony, issued a pastoral letter opposing the creation of health clinics at three high schools there. He wrote that "by making contraceptives readily available, the clinics' personnel will tacitly promote sexual relations outside of marriage." In spite of the Church's opposition, the health centers opened, and an overwhelming percentage of parents signed the consent forms. Indeed, the bickering in several cities created something of a backlash in the broader public health community. Even Republican President George H.W. Bush's Advisory Council on Social Security in 1991 sought to expand school-based clinics.[4]

By then, the nature of the debate was changing. For one thing, the team of outside evaluators that looked at the Foundation-funded clinics in 1993 found that although the new centers had greatly increased access to health care for urban youth, they had not reduced either risky behavior by teenagers, including unprotected sexual activity, or the rates of adolescent pregnancy. In fact, unmarried American teen pregnancy rates had peaked around 1990, in part because widespread publicity about AIDS had led to more condom use. But because of a normal lag in statistical data and because rates were still close to the historical highs, alarm over the problem was still high.

Those who were active in the public health community, including officials at the Robert Wood Johnson Foundation, were eager to avoid the highly divisive aspects of the teen pregnancy debate. Paul Jellinek, who was a vice president of the Foundation for much of the 1990s, said that although the Foundation continued to address ways to offer and improve health care in urban school settings, there was, by the middle of the decade, little enthusiasm for projects that tackled teen pregnancy directly. "The political problems had a lot to do with it. You had the Eagle Forum"—another socially conservative group opposing sex counseling in schools—"and the Catholic Church."

By then, policymakers in Washington were already talking about a new way to approach the issue.

A Defining Moment

A defining moment in the evolution of teen pregnancy prevention as a national issue took place on the night of January 24, 1995, when then-President Bill Clinton delivered his third State of the Union Address. Just two years into his presidency, Clinton, a Democrat, had received a resounding rebuke from voters, who had given Republicans control of both houses of Congress for the first time in decades. And so his more-than-nine-thousand-word speech focused heavily on finding centrist approaches to thorny political problems and on what he called "a new social compact" with America. In doing so, the President called special attention to some social issues that had rarely or never been discussed in such a high-profile forum—most notably teenage pregnancy.

"We've got to ask our community leaders and all kinds of organizations to help us stop our most serious social problem: the epidemic of teen pregnancies and births where there is no marriage," Clinton said. "I have sent to Congress a plan to target schools all over this country with antipregnancy programs that work. But government can only do so much. Tonight I call on parents and leaders all across this country to join together in a national campaign against teen pregnancy to make a difference. We can do this and we must."

For the White House, this was clearly seen as an issue where good politics and good government intersected. Clinton had frequently preached that America should find a centrist "third way" of resolving the most divisive social issues. What is more, he was also working to fulfill a pledge from his 1992 presidential campaign to "end welfare as we know it," and as his aides and the new GOP majority in Congress negotiated a welfare reform bill, it became clear that reducing teen pregnancy would attack poverty at its very roots and thus make it easier for policy makers facing otherwise tough choices on curbing the welfare rolls.

William Galston, now a public policy professor at the University of Maryland, was deputy assistant to the president for domestic policy during the first Clinton administration, and he took part in the White House discussions leading up to the launching of the campaign. He said the early discussions on what would become the National Campaign to Prevent Teen Pregnancy (of which he became a founding board member) were intimately wrapped into the lobbying for welfare reform. "There was a real sense that reducing the rate of teen pregnancy also has a significant impact on the welfare system, which was seen as out of control during this period," Galston said.

Another important person in those early discussions was Isabel Sawhill, who was then associate director in the Office of Management and Budget and is today the president of the National Campaign. She had been studying and observing the link between poverty and teen pregnancy since 1973, when she wrote her first book, *Time of Transition: The Growth of Families Headed by Women.* "The data are clear: the driving force behind the growth of single-parent families is now unwed births," Sawhill said recently. "And half of first unwed births are to teens. And a very high proportion of the families so formed are poor. Thus, it seemed obvious to me that if you wanted to reduce poverty you needed to reduce teen pregnancies and births."

Those discussions—and the political zeitgeist of the mid-1990s—led to what everyone involved agrees was a critical decision. This national effort, while carrying the full support and backing of the Clinton White House, would be spearheaded not by another presidential task force but by a newly created, outside nonprofit group. Most important, this national campaign would not be nonpartisan merely in name but would be aggressively bipartisan in its approach.

The tone was set in February 1996 when the chairman of the new National Campaign to Prevent Teen Pregnancy was introduced: a Republican, former New Jersey Governor Tom Kean. Like Clinton, Kean, who today is board chairman of the Robert Wood Johnson Foundation, is also a centrist on social issues and a supporter of abortion rights, and his involvement sent a powerful message to those seeking to bridge the ideological divide on teen-pregnancy prevention that had so polarized the debate during the 1980s and early 1990s.

Sarah Brown, who had been a senior study director at the Institute of Medicine, where she led numerous projects in maternal and child health, has been the executive director of the National Campaign to Prevent Teen

Pregnancy from its inception. She said that the push to include not only Kean but also other prominent Republicans with more conservative social views, such as former Minnesota congressman Vin Weber (a founding board member), was just one way that this new effort looked to change the framework of the once-gridlocked debate. Perhaps more important, she noted, was an effort to include prominent Americans from a number of fields who, prior to the 1990s, would have been unlikely candidates for a teen pregnancy prevention drive.

"In 1996, the only people who talked much about teen pregnancy prevention were people in the so-called reproductive health field, and that field is generally very progressive and very liberal," Brown said. Fairly or not, groups that had long been working for an increased emphasis on family planning, such as Planned Parenthood, seemed to have the effect of waving a red flag in front of social conservatives, and that often led to a stifled political debate. The National Campaign to Prevent Teen Pregnancy sought a much broader base. That included prominent business leaders, including the then-board chairmen of Procter & Gamble and General Mills; media executives such as the publisher of the *Washington Post* Katherine Graham and Warner Bros. TV executive Bruce Rosenblum; civil rights leader and former ambassador to the United Nations Andrew Young; and religious leader Sister Mary Rose McGeady, the president of the Catholic social-services group Covenant House.

This new, consensus-seeking approach was viewed favorably at the Robert Wood Johnson Foundation. Beginning with an initial $1.5 million grant awarded in 1996, the Foundation has provided more than $5 million in grants to the Campaign.

Rush Russell, a former Foundation senior program officer who participated in the internal discussions about the initial grant, said there had been a fair amount of debate about the first grant for the Campaign. "Teen pregnancy was not a part of the Foundation's priorities," he noted. However, Russell said, the 1992 riots in Los Angeles had prompted a new round of discussion about programs for the urban poor, and ultimately the Foundation decided that the new Campaign could be integrated into its programs targeting "vulnerable populations."

In announcing the kickoff of the Campaign in February of 1996, the fledgling organization's leaders set an extremely ambitious measurable goal:

to reduce the teen pregnancy rate in America by one-third in less than a decade, or by 2005. The Campaign set out to accomplish this by what it calls "a top-down, bottom-up strategy"; that is, it would run no direct community programs itself but instead operate both as a clearinghouse for the best data and practices on reducing teen pregnancy and as a vehicle for influencing both the entertainment media and the public debate.

For Sarah Brown, the challenges facing the National Campaign to Prevent Teen Pregnancy were driven home one night not long after it had opened its office, at 1776 Massachusetts Avenue in Washington, D.C. "I was brand new, and the phone rang and it was a guy from Cloverdale, California," said Brown. "He said that he was active in a community group and that 'We want to do something about teen pregnancy, but we don't know what to do.' And that is the question: What do you do?"

The Campaign quickly crafted an approach that in some ways could also serve as a model for advocacy groups involved with other important but socially divisive public health issues. Here are some of those principles:

Broaden the Debate

With founding board members Sawhill and Galston bringing an economics perspective, the Campaign placed a strong emphasis from its very beginning on the strong relationship between unwanted births and child poverty, with the accompanying strains on the welfare system, high crime rates, poor school systems, and child abuse. One of the Campaign's first publications was a short document called *Why It Matters,* which highlighted the negative economic and social impact of America's high rate of teenage pregnancy.

That theme has remained a fundamental principle of the Campaign to this day. In 2006, the Campaign published an ambitious report entitled *By the Numbers: The Public Costs of Teen Childbearing,* which sought to quantify the impact on American taxpayers. The report, written by the University of Delaware economics professor Saul Hoffman, found that teen childbearing cost local, state, and federal taxpayers at least $9.1 billion in 2004, the last year for which statistics were available.[5] In addition, the report breaks out the costs by all fifty states, with taxpayers in Texas bearing the heaviest burden—more than $1 billion in 2004.

Such numbers are important to the Campaign's broader goal of convincing lawmakers at the state as well the federal level of the importance of teen pregnancy prevention. The community groups said that they had various needs, according to Brown, among them "things like how do you go to your state legislator and explain why he or she should care about teenage pregnancy." Another Campaign publication, geared at lawmakers and opinion leaders, is entitled *Not Just Another Single Issue: Teen Pregnancy Prevention's Link to Other Critical Social Issues.* The Campaign's constant emphasis on the shared social costs help to shift some of the debate away from value-based issues like sex education, which proved so acrimonious.

Find Common Ground

By the time that the Campaign was launched, in 1996, there was already a strong movement under way for abstinence education in public schools, including so-called abstinence-only programs that encouraged young people to avoid sex altogether as the only way to prevent pregnancy and other unwanted consequences. Although such programs are associated with the conservative movement that elected Ronald Reagan in the 1980s and George W. Bush in the 2000s, in fact, the federal government dramatically increased federal funding of abstinence programs during the Clinton administration. In 1996, as Clinton was seeking re-election, and having promised voters he would "end welfare as we know it," he ultimately signed a version of legislation that included a measure drafted in the Republican-controlled Congress, which included $50 million in federal grants for state and local abstinence programs, to be matched with more than $40 million of local spending.

When the Campaign began that same year, its leaders determined that the group would seek to work with the abstinence-only movement. Ironically, the Campaign adopted a popular term from Republican politics, calling the model a "big-tent" approach. The concept, according to Campaign officials, was that no effort that could play a positive role of any kind toward reducing teen pregnancy rate should be shunned. The board's Bill Galston came to call this approach "Unity of goal, diversity of means."

Obtain and Disseminate Reliable Information

Another way that the Campaign steers clear of political divisiveness is by taking approaches based as much as possible on scientific data. What that means, according to those involved, is finding, digesting, and then promulgating the best available research on both what social factors promote teen pregnancy and what methods work best to reduce them. The Campaign disseminates this data extensively to local groups that can use it in their own efforts.

"I think that one of the critical things, and one of our foundations, is that you've got to get your facts straight," Brown said. "A lot of people who fight over things, when you dig around, you find that they're really rooted in ideology." Instead, she said, the Campaign tries to seek out the best ideas, regardless of whether they support or contradict the conventional wisdom on teen pregnancy, and put them to use.

One of the Campaign's most widely used efforts has been a section on its Web site, as well as in its printed documents, with the simple title *What Works.* Recently, the Campaign boiled down some of its findings over the last decade into a nineteen-page *What Works* pamphlet for school administrators and community activists. In clear language, the pamphlet lays out the types of programs that have been most successful in reducing a locality's teen pregnancy rate. These include curriculum-based programs that discuss both abstinence and contraception as well as broader programs that target academics and career and job development for teenagers, like the one in New Britain, Connecticut. The campaign's Web site also includes features such as a scientific analysis of how some four hundred different factors affect teen sexual behavior, as well as the latest research showing that children of teen parents are less prepared upon entering school.[6] The Campaign's Web site received more than eleven million visits between 2000 and 2006.

Reach Out to the Media and Parents

One area in which the Campaign has elected to play a direct role has been in dealing with the nation's media. The naming of the *Washington Post*'s Graham and Warner Bros.' Rosenblum to its board was just the start of the effort to develop closer ties with the big media companies based in Hollywood and in New York.

The Campaign has actively sought to involve itself in plot lines of TV shows and on the pages of magazines popular for youth. For example, between the late-1990s and mid-2006, it forged a close tie with *Teen People,* a now-defunct magazine published by Time, Inc. The magazine published a number of articles concerning teen pregnancy prevention, including a two-page color spread of attractive and athletic teens with the headline "Can You Spot the Virgin?" (It was a trick question: they were all virgins.)

Like other public-interest groups, the Campaign has produced a number of public-service announcements aimed at a teen audience. But one thing that set its efforts apart has been its efforts to alter the content of the types of television shows and movies that have always glamorized sex but rarely showed the potential real-life consequences of an unplanned pregnancy.

In 1998, for example, the Campaign worked closely with the ABC soap opera *One Life to Live* to incorporate a story line about a teenage girl who didn't use contraception the first time she had sex—and became pregnant. The story line, which lasted the entire nine months of the pregnancy, was later boiled down to a ten-minute video and study guide distributed to some ten thousand schools and community groups. The Campaign worked with ABC again in 2006 on a similar story line on *General Hospital,* which was based in part on talking points drafted by the organization.[7]

Research established that messages from the mass media were very important, as was the role of peers—and of parents. Ironically, parents had often been excluded from the discussion, partly because the family-planning-oriented programs of 1970s and 1980s were built on a belief that sexually active teens would not ask for contraceptives if parents knew more about such programs.

"There was more of a focus on simply getting contraceptives to teenagers," said Judith E. Jones, a pioneer in the movement who is a clinical professor at the Mailman School of Public Health at Columbia University and serves on the Campaign's board of directors. "Most people felt that parents shouldn't be involved—that kids would not get contraceptives." Today, the Campaign not only encourages parents to talk to their teenage children about avoiding pregnancy but also promotes its *Ten Tips for Parents to Help Their Children Avoid Teen Pregnancy.*

Reasons for the Decline in Teen Pregnancy

A variety of new statistics and studies have made it clear that the initial ten-year push of the Campaign has coincided with an unprecedented drop in pregnancies and births to unmarried teenagers in America. The Campaign's target was a one-third reduction, and the most recent available government statistics analyzed by the Guttmacher Institute show that teen pregnancy rates declined by 36 percent between 1990 and 2002.[8] The reduction among black teenagers, who had been targeted by many locally based efforts, was even larger, at 40 percent.

What is responsible for this trend? At the most basic level, the way to reduce teen pregnancy is either through less sexual activity or through increased or more effective contraception. The most in-depth study of this question, a recently published study by a team led by John Santelli, a professor at the Mailman School of Public Health, Columbia University and a senior fellow at the Guttmacher Institute, found that although the picture is a mixed one; the largest share of the decline in teen pregnancy is attributable to both increased and better use of contraceptives. The researchers concluded that about 86 percent of the decline is the result of contraceptive practices, with a revealing difference when teenagers are separated into a younger and an older age bracket. Among the eighteen- and nineteen-year-olds surveyed, contraception accounted for almost all of the drop. Among fifteen- to seventeen-year-olds, the study found that contraceptives accounted for 77 percent, meaning that abstinence, which accounted for the remaining 23 percent, also played a significant role for this age group.[9]

The debate over abstinence versus contraception fails to answer a critical question: What were the underlying social factors that caused teenagers to increase contraception use or defer sexual activity during this period of declining rates in the 1990s and early 2000s? It appears that a number of factors came into play at the same time that, when taken all together, had a positive impact. Those factors included the following:

- *Greater awareness and concern among teenagers about contracting HIV/AIDS and other sexually transmitted diseases* throughout the 1990s, which in turn led to increased use of condoms and also lowered the pregnancy rate. The Santelli-led study found that in the seven years from 1995 to 2002 condom use among teenagers who were sexually active increased from 36 percent to 53 percent, and the improvement was more pronounced in the fifteen-to-seventeen-year-old group. What's more, better education about the effectiveness of condoms in preventing HIV/AIDS led to a much larger number of teens using two contraceptives at the same time, such as condoms and birth control pills—with a positive impact on pregnancy rates.
- *Technological improvements in contraception.* For example, the 1990s saw increasing use of Depo-Provera, a form of contraception that can be given in three-month injections as opposed to a birth control pill that must be taken daily. The rate of Depo-Provera use is highest in the United States among black teenagers, in part because of its free availability in inner-city health clinics. Its rate of effectiveness is dramatically better than that of other available methods.
- *The federal welfare reform program that was enacted in 1996,* the same year that the Campaign was founded, and came into effect by the end of the decade. The 1996 law included a requirement that teen mothers under the age of eighteen live with their parents or in another supervised setting and remain in school. Also, a number of states enacted provisions to deny additional benefits for a second child who was born or conceived while the mother was already receiving welfare. So far, academic researchers are divided over how much these law changes have affected teen behavior, but community activists—like New Britain's Bilodeau, for example—believe welfare reform is a factor. "Personally, I

think welfare reform has a lot to do with the reductions," she said.

- *Changing social mores.* The evidence of declining sexual activity by high school-aged teens is clearly a factor in the decline in teen pregnancy, although it is difficult for researchers to quantify how much of the drop is the result of fear of HIV/AIDS; how much because of abstinence-only education, boosted by the sharp rise in federal funding of it since the enactment of welfare reform; and how much is simply due to a more conservative social climate among American teenagers and their parents. At the Campaign, Sarah Brown noted that the most recent public opinion surveys show that not only most parents but a majority of teenagers themselves support the concept of teens delaying sexual activity until they are older, and she called this "one of five or six contributing factors" in reducing rates.

Campaign officials readily acknowledge that it is impossible to place a hard statistical value on the role that its own efforts have played in the pregnancy-rate reduction, although they believe they deserve some measure of credit. A number of experts who study teen pregnancy agree with them. The Campaign contracts with the consulting firm McKinsey & Company to evaluate its effectiveness and also uses national public opinion surveys to gauge how and how much teen sexual practices and mores are changing.

In August 2003, McKinsey delivered the results of a survey of the people the campaign considers its "customers," a list that includes policy leaders—state and local officials as well as journalists and entertainment executives. More than 80 percent of those in the teen pregnancy prevention field reported that the Campaign had helped them to be more effective in their work.

McKinsey also found that its clients in each of the categories listed the Campaign as the primary resource among a dozen groups that dealt with teen pregnancy issues. Using another measure, in a viewer survey after the consumer giant General Mills worked with the WB Network, now the CW Network, to incorporate a teen pregnancy awareness message into the popular series *Dawson's Creek,* 68 percent of viewers aged thirteen to seventeen said the shows made them more aware of the risks and consequences of sex.

Other Programs Funded by the Robert Wood Johnson Foundation

The Robert Wood Johnson Foundation has also supported a number of smaller and midsized teen pregnancy prevention programs. Not surprisingly, these programs have also reflected a mix of strategies, with some that stress abstinence and others that emphasize a range of preventive measures, including contraceptives.

In fact, even before the launch of the Campaign, the Foundation had supported an early abstinence-based program, the Washington, D.C.-based Best Friends Foundation, which had been created in response to a rising inner-city teen pregnancy rate during the 1980s by Elayne Bennett, a Georgetown University educator who is also the wife of former U.S. Secretary of Education William Bennett. The youth development program for girls in grades six through twelve seeks to promote abstinence in sexual activity, drinking, smoking, and using drugs by raising self-esteem among the girls though a combination of mentoring and strong role models, as well as participation in cultural activities like music and dance.

From 1990 through 2003, the Foundation awarded a total of $2.2 million in five grants to the Best Friends Foundation, beginning with a small pilot project in Washington and growing in the mid-1990s with funding to help expand the model into more than half a dozen other school systems across the country. The relationship between the Foundation and the Best Friends Foundation hit a snag, however, with a disagreement over the best way to evaluate the abstinence program. When the Best Friends group could not agree on an evaluation plan with the Foundation-hired evaluators, Mathematica Policy Research of Princeton, New Jersey, the Foundation's support of the program was gradually phased out.[10] [11]

For the most part, the other teen pregnancy reduction efforts financed by Foundation grants have tended to be smaller, community-based programs that take a comprehensive approach that includes access to contraception but centers on education—not just about relationships or the risk of sexually transmitted disease but also about career training and academics. Overall, the Foundation has spent roughly $5 million since the early 1980s on these smaller programs, as well as for opinion research and scientific study on teen pregnancy prevention.

One program in the Foundation's backyard, funded through the Foundation's New Jersey Health Initiatives program, is a school-based pregnancy prevention effort at three schools in Atlantic County in the south-central part of the state. In 1999, the Foundation awarded $270,000 to Atlantic County for three schools to launch an offshoot of a program called Teen Choice, which appeared to be effective in the far different, urban environs of upper Manhattan. The program, which is not connected to other Foundation-supported programs like the Campaign, was launched after statistics showed Atlantic County had among the highest teen birth rates in New Jersey.

One of the three schools was Buena Regional High School in Buena, New Jersey, a rural community where many parents commute to service jobs in the Atlantic City casinos, about forty minutes away. Just as at the Pathway/Senderos program in New Britain, a visitor to Teen Choice at Buena High at first might not realize he was witnessing a program dealing with teen pregnancy. At one session on a Tuesday morning, about forty students filed into an airy, cinder-block school library to watch a series of skits performed by a group of their peers—acting students from a technical high school in neighboring Burlington County, New Jersey. The skits, and even a musical number, centered on the theme of domestic violence in long-term relationships and toward gays.

In one skit, a girl delivered a soliloquy to her baby brother about calling in protective services to deal with their physically abusive mom, while in another, an African-American recounted her relationship with the white father of her child as he became drawn toward skinhead politics and the couple descends into violence and abuse. The racially mixed group of Buena students applauded the sometimes emotionally jarring production. Its message about healthy relationships, while indirect, is increasingly a major part of pregnancy prevention programs.

Kathy Bress, the program's coordinator since it began in 1999, said the skits fit well with the program's broader goals of boosting self-esteem as well as healthy teen relationships. The Teen Choice program also places a strong emphasis on peer-to-peer counseling, through what it calls a natural helpers program. Bress herself also works hard to build close ties with students, attending their sporting events and other activities "so they just don't think of you as 'the sex lady.'"

Yet in many ways the Teen Choice program is rooted in some of the highly traditional norms of teen pregnancy prevention. Although community leaders do not permit the distribution of condoms, the school-based program is aggressive in sending sexually active students to family-planning clinics. "There isn't a bus that comes through here, so we really have to negotiate time to get them to the facilities," Bress explained.

The Future

In May 2005, the National Campaign to Prevent Teen Pregnancy celebrated its tenth anniversary by announcing that it was setting an equally ambitious goal for its second decade: to reduce the rate of teenage pregnancy by another one-third by the year 2015. Campaign officials conceded that reaching the target would require new approaches to build on the basic strategy developed during the 1990s.

"I don't know whether it's realistic, but it's good to set a goal that will challenge the country as well as the organization to do better," said Isabel Sawhill, the Campaign's president. Officials note that despite the dramatic reductions of the last ten years, teen pregnancy and birth rates in the United States remain much higher than in the other industrialized nations.

Thus, Campaign officials are looking more closely at factors in teen pregnancy that had not been emphasized in earlier successful programs. One of these is the role that young men and teenage boys play in preventing unwanted pregnancies. A February 2006 report released by the campaign entitled *It's a Guy Thing: Boys, Young Men and Teen Pregnancy Prevention* noted that, with little fanfare, reduced sexual activity and increased condom use driven by male behavior had accounted for some of the recent drop in pregnancy rates; it encouraged local programs to work more closely with males to accelerate this trend.

Brown said that although her group has always worked closely with religious leaders, the Campaign is currently increasing its efforts to learn more about the role that a person's faith and belief system can play in efforts to reduce pregnancy, mainly by promoting abstinence. It is also focusing more on how issues like sexual abuse affect teenage behavior, and thus pregnancy.

But officials acknowledge that future funding is a concern. At the Campaign itself, Brown said she is worried about what she called "issues fatigue" as donors and activists look toward newer issues in the public spotlight. There is also the lingering impact of the current administration in Washington, which restricts most federal funding for teen pregnancy prevention to abstinence-only programs. Currently, the Campaign is on its fifth grant from the Robert Wood Johnson Foundation—funding that ends January 2008. In May of 2007, Campaign officials announced that it was expanding its core mission to include an effort to reduce unwanted pregnancies among women in their twenties and older, with the help of a three-year, $18-million grant from the William and Flora Hewlett Foundation. The effort is a response, they said, to new data showing that unwanted pregnancies among older women have not declined at the same rate as they have for teenagers.

Regardless of whether its ambitious new goal of reducing teen pregnancies by one-third can be reached, officials said the Campaign has already provided a kind of road map for how society can tackle its most politically divisive public health problems—with good science and best practices at the core, but also a willingness to listen to and work within the broad range of American cultural, religious, and community standards, as well as understanding the role of media in shaping opinions.

Notes

1. Jones, E. F., and others. *Teenage Pregnancy in Industrialized Countries.* New Haven: Yale University Press, 1986.
2. Congressional Budget Office. *Sources of Support for Adolescent Mothers.* Washington, D.C.: Congress, Feb. 1990.
3. Brodeur, P. "School Based Health Clinics." *To Improve Health and Health Care 2000: The Robert Wood Johnson Foundation Anthology.* San Francisco: Jossey-Bass, 2000, 3–33.
4. Ibid.

5. Hoffman, S. "By the Numbers: The Public Costs of Teen Childbearing." National Campaign to Prevent Teen Pregnancy, October 2006. (http://www.teenpregnancy.org/costs/default.asp)
6. National Campaign to Prevent Teen Pregnancy. "What Works." (http://www.teenpregnancy.org/resources/reading/pdf/What_Works.pdf)
7. Reimer, S. "Teen Pregnancy Story Line on Soap Opera Tackles Some Real-Life Issues." *Baltimore Sun,* Aug. 27, 2006.
8. The Guttmacher Institute. *U.S. Teenage Pregnancy Statistics National and State Trends and Trends by Race and Ethnicity.* New York: The Guttmacher Institute, 2006.
9. Santelli, J. S., and others. "Explaining Recent Declines in Adolescent Pregnancy in the United States: The Contribution of Abstinence and Contraceptive Use." *American Journal of Public Health, 2007, 97(1) 150–156.*
10. Robert Wood Johnson Foundation. Multi-State "Best Friends" Program Prevents Risky Behaviors Among Teenage Girls. Robert Wood Johnson Foundation Grant Results Report, May 2005. (http://www.rwjf.org/portfolios/resources/grants report.jsp?filename=029684.htm&iaid=144&gsa=1)
11. A study of two thousand children in federally funded abstinence-only programs by Mathematica Policy Research, released in April 2007, found that these programs were ineffective. The report stated that young people in the programs "were no more likely to abstain from sex than their control group counterparts." (http://www.mathematica-mpr.com/publications/PDFs/impactabstinence.pdf)

CHAPTER 4

The Smoke-Free Families Program

Fen Montaigne

Editors' Introduction

Tobacco remains the leading cause of preventable deaths in the United States. Since 1991, the Robert Wood Johnson Foundation has given high priority to reducing smoking, expending more than $142 million on a wide range of tobacco-control activities. The Foundation's efforts were singled out by Joel Fleishman in his book, *The Foundation: A Great American Secret,* as one of twelve foundation-driven initiatives that have achieved high impact.[1]

Previous volumes of the Anthology have featured ten chapters on the Foundation's tobacco-control work.[2] In this chapter, Fen Montaigne examines a single program, Smoke-Free Families, which was designed to find ways to help pregnant smokers quit. Set in the context of a clinical guideline issued by the United States Public Health Service recommending ways (called the 5 A's) that physicians can help their patients stop smoking, the Smoke-Free Families program funded research on counseling techniques and other ways to motivate pregnant women to stop smoking; demonstration programs to test apparently effective methods; and broad dissemination of methods that have been shown to be workable, so that they become a standard component of prenatal care.

Fen Montaigne, the author of this chapter and a former writer for the *Philadelphia Inquirer,* is a freelance journalist specializing in science and the environment. Montaigne's work has appeared in *Smithsonian, Forbes,* and *Audubon* magazines, as well as the *Wall Street Journal.* He is currently working on a book about global warming and its effect on Antarctica.

Notes

1. Fleishman, J. L. *The Foundation: A Great American Secret.* New York: Public Affairs Press, 2007.
2. See Bornemeier, J. "Taking on Tobacco: The Robert Wood Johnson Foundation's Assault on Tobacco." *To Improve Health and Health Care, Vol. VIII: The Robert Wood Johnson Foundation Anthology.* San Francisco: Jossey-Bass, 2005, for a synopsis of Foundation-funded tobacco-control programs.

—m— Zachary Bechtol is a family physician in Grove, Oklahoma, a town of 5,700 people situated on Grand Lake O' the Cherokees in the northeastern corner of the state. The breadth of his practice—Bechtol does everything from colonoscopies to cesarean sections—might come as a surprise to family practitioners in major metropolitan areas. But in rural Delaware County, which borders Arkansas and Missouri, a general practitioner must master many medical arts. His range recalls an era depicted by Norman Rockwell in his portraits of family doctors, but the similarity ends there: Bechtol, thirty-eight, is a fit, handsome, straight-talking physician who scrambles to make a good living and deliver top-notch treatment in an age of unbridled litigation and managed care.

Bechtol is known both in the region and at the University of Oklahoma's Department of Family and Preventive Medicine in Oklahoma City as a doctor interested in bringing the latest therapies into his practice. He is a member of the Oklahoma Physicians Research/Resource Network, a group of 230 practitioners in ninety locations that participates in research projects and translates them into action. But even Bechtol would acknowledge that he was falling short in one area: how to help smokers—particularly pregnant smokers—kick their cigarette addiction. And so, in early 2004, when he heard through the research network about a program to teach physicians and nurses how to more effectively counsel and help pregnant smokers, he was eager to participate.

The program was known as Smoke-Free Beginnings, a pilot project funded under the Robert Wood Johnson Foundation's Smoke-Free Families initiative. Begun in 1994 and funded through August of 2008, Smoke-Free Families was designed to support research into effective ways to help pregnant smokers quit, test those methods in a series of demonstration projects, and encourage their incorporation into everyday prenatal care. The idea was to ensure that physicians across the country would use the latest tools to sharply reduce smoking among pregnant women, which is the leading preventable cause of low-birthweight babies, preterm deliveries, and perinatal death. The program, which has spent more than $23 million on research and disseminating its findings, also targeted postpartum mothers so that their babies would not suffer the ill effects of secondhand smoke.

For Bechtol, participation in Smoke-Free Beginnings meant that the project coordinator, Sarah Jane Carlson, and a staff member from the Oklahoma Physicians Research/Resource Network regularly visited the office to coach Bechtol and his nurses in counseling techniques. The evidence-based techniques are known as the "5 A's"—ask, advise, assess, assist, and arrange—and they have been shown to significantly increase the quit rate of pregnant smokers.

The 5 A's

In 2000, the United States Public Health Service issued a Clinical Practice Guideline, *Treating Tobacco Use and Dependence,* recommending that practitioners treat patients who smoke using the 5 A's brief intervention. The 5 A's are:

- *Ask* patients about their tobacco use at every visit and document findings.
- *Advise* them to quit in a clear, strong, and personalized manner.
- *Assess* their willingness to attempt to quit within the next thirty days.
- *Assist* those individuals willing to attempt to quit using counseling and, unless it is contraindicated, pharmacotherapy.
- *Arrange* appropriate follow-up.[1]

The Guideline recommended a more intensive approach to address the special needs of pregnant women—the augmented 5 A's. Instead of the normal two-to-three-minute counseling given to nonpregnant smokers, the panel suggested that pregnant women be asked specific questions about their smoking status, receive five to fifteen minutes of behavioral counseling, and be given pregnancy-specific self-help materials. Noting that cessation medications had not been recommended as safe or effective for routine use in pregnancy, due to possible harm to the fetus, it advised clinicians to carefully weigh the risks and benefits of their potential use. The augmented 5 A's practice is recommended by the American College of Obstetricians and Gynecologists and the U.S. Public Health Service, among others.

To make the augmented 5 A's a routine part of office visits for pregnant patients, Carlson's team urged Bechtol and his staff to use a brightly colored piece of paper, known as a flow sheet, that contained detailed questions about a pregnant smoker's habit and attempts to quit. The 5 A's for all smokers are based on a cardinal rule of smoking cessation counseling: the more a doctor, nurse, or counselor talks with a smoker about his or her addiction and spells out techniques for quitting, the greater the likelihood that a smoker will give up cigarettes. As Michael Fiore, a physician who founded the University of Wisconsin Center for Tobacco Research and a leading tobacco-control expert who chaired the panel that wrote the 2000 Public Health Service Guideline, put it, "What we know about smoking cessation counseling is that it's a clear dose-response effect: the more minutes spent with the smoker, the higher the quit rate." With doubts about the appropriateness of medication for pregnant women, counseling is recommended as first-line treatment for expectant mothers.

Like many obstetrician/gynecologists, Bechtol had been asking his pregnant patients if they smoked and had urged the smokers to quit. But neither he nor his staff had been trained in the art of counseling, nor had they been spending sufficient time referring pregnant smokers to resources such as Oklahoma's free telephone quitline. Eileen Merchen, a practice enhancement assistant (PEA) from the Physicians Research Network who worked with Smoke-Free Beginnings, said of Bechtol, "He was just busy, busy, busy. He'd tend to want to say directly, 'Quit eating so much' or 'Stop smoking,' and so we worked with him on counseling and having more empathy with the patients."

Bechtol began applying the techniques taught by Merchen and Carlson to the sixty to seventy pregnant patients he saw annually, about a quarter of whom smoked. That is higher than the national smoking rate for pregnant women, which is estimated to range between 12 and 22 percent.[2] About three-quarters of his pregnant patients are covered by Medicaid and most have not attended college.

"Smoking is huge here—it's part of the culture," said Bechtol, who—dressed in blue jeans and a blue down vest—spoke on a Friday afternoon after seeing patients. "You can't be judgmental. You have to be on their side. You're treating these women during one of life's most stressful situations, which is having a baby. More than half the women I take care of are unwed, and all of a sudden you want to take away one of the most reliable things to them—their cigarette. But I say, 'Hey, you're the mama. You get to decide if the baby is going to be healthy.' You try to get them to understand that if they have a low-birthweight baby born at thirty or thirty-two weeks, they'll be spending a lot of time in the pediatric intensive-care unit in Tulsa. You get people to where they want to talk about it. We try to make a difference one pregnant person at a time."

Bechtol was able to incorporate the 5 A's into his office's hectic routine because the counseling could be accomplished quickly, and the flow-sheets and prominently placed smoking-cessation guides prompted him and his staff to pursue the smoking issue. "They helped us systematize this," Bechtol recalled. "You've got to take the doctor's memory out of the equation. So now things are done automatically at the beginning of a visit. You take blood pressure and temperature and you ask about their smoking."

Tanya Jackson, a thirty-two-year-old lab technician in Bechtol's office who also helps counsel pregnant smokers, said that Smoke-Free Beginnings had given her the awareness—and the skills—to talk to the expectant mothers effectively.

"Smoke-Free Beginnings empowered us and gave us the tools," Jackson said. "We'd ask them how long they had been smoking and see if a certain home situation was causing them to smoke. We'd help them set quit dates. We had pamphlets with lots of information about what would happen to their baby if they smoked during pregnancy. We'd give them the quitline number. We would be a sounding board. When they'd say, 'I can't quit because my husband smokes,' we were there to listen. If they continued smoking, then every visit during their pregnancy we'd really try to get them to quit smoking. And postpartum, if they relapsed, we'd ask them why they thought they had relapsed. Was it the stress of the newborn or a situation at home? And we'd always get Dr. Bechtol to come in and counsel, too. I feel like it's had an impact. I'd say that after counseling, 15 to 20 percent of the smokers quit."

One pregnant smoker whom Bechtol and his staff successfully reached was Piper Hall. In 2004, at age twenty-four, she was pregnant with her second daughter. The previous year, Hall had smoked throughout her first pregnancy, although she did cut down from two packs to about ten cigarettes a day. She was then under the care of a different doctor, who did not aggressively press Hall to jettison her cigarette habit, for the simple reason that she had recently kicked an addiction to methamphetamines. "I'd been using meth every day," recalled Hall, who now lives in Grove with her parents and two girls, Jade, three, and Riley, two. "I quit cold turkey."

Pregnant a second time, and now on her own as a single parent, she still smoked when she began going to Dr. Bechtol. "I went in there and I was not even thinking about my smoking and he said that if I wanted to quit, he could help," said Hall, who is returning to college to study real estate. "He talked to me for about ten minutes about why I should quit. We discussed the health effects on the baby. My first girl was born in perfect health. I got very, very lucky. I knew smoking wasn't a good thing, and so him bringing it up was all I needed. So the next day I quit. It needed to be done."

The Origins of Smoke-Free Families

Piper Hall's story is a vivid example of what the Smoke-Free Families program helped accomplish in its dozen years of existence. In the early 1990s, under the leadership of the Robert Wood Johnson Foundation's third president, Steven Schroeder, and vice president Nancy Kaufman, the Foundation made an enormous commitment to reducing smoking in the United States. From 1994 through 2006, it spent more than $600 million on a variety of tobacco-control initiatives. One of the earliest of these, and the first to focus on cessation, was Smoke-Free Families: Innovations to Stop Smoking During and Beyond Pregnancy, which has been one the Foundation's longest and most highly funded tobacco-control programs.

Targeting pregnant smokers was a natural step for the Foundation. Not only had it funded programs to reduce infant mortality and low-birthweight babies, but it also realized that many expectant mothers might well be willing to try to give up smoking in order to protect the health of their babies. Just as smoking overall was, and is, the leading cause of preventable death in the United States—smoking kills more than four hundred thousand Americans a year and accounts for more than $167 billion annually in preventable health care costs and lost productivity—so, too, is smoking the major preventable cause of perinatal complications and deaths.[3] On average, according to Robert Goldenberg, an obstetrician/gynecologist who for thirteen years directed the Smoke-Free Families National Program Office, babies born to smoking mothers weigh one-half to three-quarters of a pound less than babies born to nonsmoking mothers. Twenty percent of the low-birthweight babies are born to smoking mothers, and smoking accounts for 8 percent of preterm deliveries and 5 percent of perinatal deaths.[4] Among smoking's many harmful effects are the toxins it delivers, chiefly carbon monoxide and nicotine, which decrease blood flow from the mother to the fetus. The longer a woman has smoked, and the more she smokes, the greater the reduction of oxygen to the developing baby.

For this and other reasons, the impact of smoking on developing fetuses and newborns is significant. In addition to problems of low birth weight and prematurity, the harmful effects include increased risks of delayed conception and infertility, ectopic pregnancies, spontaneous abortions, placenta previa and placental abruption, congenital malformations, sudden infant death syndrome, and impacts on cognitive abilities.[5]

Another reason the Foundation established a program for pregnant smokers was the benefit of targeting members of a smoking population when they are open to the idea of quitting and are visiting physicians regularly for prenatal checkups. "Pregnant smokers are high risk, they are in frequent contact with the health care system, and they have a heightened motivation to quit," explained C. Tracy Orleans, senior scientist and distinguished fellow at the Robert Wood Johnson Foundation who was a key architect in the design of the program.

Orleans and Dianne Barker, the Robert Wood Johnson Foundation program officer for Smoke-Free Families in its first two years, initially consulted with experts from the Centers for Disease Control and Prevention and the National Institutes of Health on research needed to help pregnant smokers quit. At that time, about eight hundred thousand pregnant women in the United States smoked—roughly one-fifth of all expectant mothers in the country.

"Our early intention was to fund small studies to see if we could find interventions to push the rates of quitting beyond what they were at the time," said Barker, who also served as chairwoman of the Smoke-Free Families national advisory council and now runs Barker Bi-Coastal Health Consultants in Calabasas, California. "And the emphasis was not just on pregnant women but on pregnant women and their young families. We intentionally called the program Smoke-Free Families to emphasize that."

Orleans recalled, "Our hope was to catalyze breakthrough innovations and really increase the quit rate of pregnant women at a crucial time in their lives. We also wanted to find new ways to prevent postpartum relapse. In short, we wanted the program to be an incubator for good ideas—hoping to trigger follow-on National Institutes of Health studies of promising results and to identify effective interventions that could be widely applied."

Once the program helped develop more effective treatment approaches, Smoke-Free Families planned to spread the word to the community of obstetrician/gynecologists and family practitioners. "We saw that this gap needed to be addressed to reach an incredibly important population and with a huge return on investment," Orleans said, "We didn't have anything to show ob/gyns and say, 'If you do this it will make a huge difference.'"

In the mid-1990s, a sizable number of ob/gyns and family practitioners would ask pregnant patients if they smoked and advise them to quit. But the majority did little else.[6] There was scant impetus to do more, as private health insurers and Medicaid did not reimburse physicians for cessation counseling, and neither the federal government nor the American College of Obstetricians and Gynecologists had drafted guidelines on counseling pregnant smokers. But Smoke-Free Families was being launched at a propitious time, as tobacco cessation and control efforts were gaining momentum. Already, at the midpoint of what Pulitzer Prize-winning author Richard Kluger has labeled the "Hundred Year War" against tobacco,[7] smoking rates among the general population had dropped from a peak of 43 percent in 1955 to roughly 20 to 22 percent in the mid-1990s. Among women aged eighteen to twenty-four, smoking rates had declined from 38 percent in 1965 to 25 percent in 2000, and smoking rates among women aged twenty-five to forty-four had fallen from 44 percent to 23 percent during the same years.[8]

Tap into the memories of baby boomers and you will see how far things have come. A significant number of people born in the two decades between 1945 and the issuance of the 1964 Surgeon General's report on smoking had mothers—many of them with college degrees—who smoked during pregnancy. Today, you almost never see a pregnant, college-educated woman lighting up a cigarette. Smoking—especially among pregnant women—is now an activity largely confined to the poorer and less well educated in our society. Only two percent of college-educated women smoke, whereas 27 percent of women with a high school education do.[9] In 2000, some 25 percent of pregnant women covered by Medicaid were smokers—double the rate among the overall population of pregnant women.[10]

Smoke-Free Families: An Overview

The goal of the Smoke-Free Families initiative was to reduce smoking before, during, and after pregnancy, using a three-pronged strategy. The first was to fund research that would identify effective cessation treatments for pregnant smokers and their families. This was carried out under the auspices of the National Program Office located at the University of Alabama, Birmingham, for the first thirteen years of the project. It moved to Drexel University when Robert Goldenberg, the program's national director, relocated there in 2007.

The second prong was to fund demonstration projects to find ways to incorporate effective interventions into routine prenatal and postpartum care. Between 1994 and 2000, this was overseen by the National Program Office; in 2000, the Foundation established a National Dissemination Office to fund and oversee demonstration projects and to publicize the work being done under the Smoke-Free Families program. Located at the Cecil G. Sheps Center for Health Services Research at the University of North Carolina at Chapel Hill, the office was directed by Cathy Melvin, a leading epidemiologist whose specialty is maternal health and tobacco control.

The third prong was to promote the acceptance of the effective interventions to help pregnant and parenting smokers quit. This aspect was carried out by a coalition of influential organizations and agencies called the National Partnership to Help Pregnant Smokers Quit, or National Partnership. Established in 2002, the National Partnership is also directed by Melvin and run out of the Sheps Center at the University of North Carolina.

Research

The first phase of research grants, from 1994 to 1998, funded eleven investigations at a cost of $5.45 million. The studies were relatively small and explored a variety of approaches: from using biofeedback to show women how prevalent nicotine was in their system to testing the efficacy of using peer ex-smokers to counsel pregnant smokers. Later studies explored the use of home visits by nurses to prevent relapse among postpartum smokers and the payment of cash incentives to smokers for quitting (which was also tested in phase one).

The results of these studies were published in two widely circulated journal supplements. One of the most important conclusions from the Smoke-Free Family studies, along with other studies, was that five to fifteen minutes of counseling—the "augmented 5 A's"—for pregnant women on the first visit and subsequent visits, supplemented by pregnancy-specific self-help material, succeeded in increasing quit levels to two to three times the rate of control groups: roughly 17 percent of pregnant women receiving the augmented 5 A's counseling quit smoking, compared with a quit rate of 7 percent for women who did not receive counseling.[11]

It proved more difficult than expected to improve on the core 5 A's counseling results. The payment of cash incentives in conjunction with counseling, however, emerged as a promising exception. In one experiment in Oregon, more than 200 women participated in a study to see if those receiving a $50 monthly cash voucher that could be exchanged for baby items, as well as counseling from a trained, self-designated "significant other" supporter, led to higher quit rates. The financial incentives and counseling greatly improved quit rates: in their eighth month of pregnancy, 32 percent of the treatment group had stopped smoking, compared with 9 percent of the control group. Two months after delivery, 21 percent of the treatment group still had not resumed smoking, while only 6 percent of the control group remained tobacco-free.[12] Other studies have shown that pregnant women receiving financial incentives alone have quit rates of approximately 30 percent—two to three times higher than women who received no payments to quit smoking.[13]

Paying pregnant smokers not to do something that, out of concern for their babies, they should stop doing anyway, can be a controversial approach. Paying drug users to abstain has certainly raised controversy. But Stephen Higgins, professor of psychiatry and co-director of Substance Abuse Treatment Center at the University of Vermont, said such interventions might be necessary to reach the hard-core smokers and women who relapse after delivery. Higgins, who has done considerable research into using financial incentives with drug addicts, said the smoking cessation community had generally committed itself to a "low-intensity public health model with broad reach"—the 5 A's. But the model breaks down when it confronts the heavily addicted.

"My experience with pregnant women smokers is that many have a problem with cigarettes that is a serious problem of drug dependency," Higgins said. "They're very often young, poor, and depressed. I've worked five years with this population of women and that's long enough to know that you will not get them to quit with the 5 A's. The ones who are likely to respond to that kind of intervention are the less severely addicted and more socially stable. We are ignoring a second, more intense option that would deal with the more seriously addicted. The more I see these women, the more I think it's going to take a specialized intensive service staffed by trained professionals."

Although the use of smoking-cessation drugs can pose risks to the fetus—and for that reason was not part of the research program at all—Smoke-Free Families did commission literature reviews of the relevant research on the risks and benefits of cessation medications. This is a controversial area, with some researchers concluding that the benefits of prescribing a carefully controlled dose of nicotine (through a nicotine patch) could outweigh the risks of smoking. "Although the use of nicotine replacement products may not be completely without risk, the risk is certainly much less than that of cigarette smoke," wrote Neal L. Benowitz and Delia A. Dempsey of the Division of Clinical Pharmacology and Experimental Therapeutics at the San Francisco General Hospital Medical Center in an article published in 2004.[14] Cheryl Oncken of the University of Connecticut Health Center, reviewing the literature in 2006, suggested that great caution is needed when prescribing smoking-cessation medication—particularly nicotine patches, which deliver a constant dose of nicotine. In her presentation at the Smoke-Free Families "capstone" meeting in 2006, Oncken concluded, "No study has yet established the safety or efficacy of the use of any of the pharmacotherapeutic smoking-cessation treatments during pregnancy." The safety and effectiveness of cessation medications for pregnant and breastfeeding women is one of the topics that will be examined in the 2008 update of the current 2000 clinical practice guideline.

Another finding of the research underwritten by Smoke-Free Families was the extent to which pregnant women conceal the fact that they smoke: in one study, up to 23 percent of pregnant women covered by Medicaid denied that they smoked, as did 14 percent of women insured by private companies. Such findings have helped researchers and physicians devise a more nuanced method of asking pregnant women about their smoking than requesting a simple "yes" or "no." These questionnaires, which ask women, for example, if they still smoke but have cut down since becoming pregnant, elicit more far more truthful responses.

Demonstration Projects and Dissemination

After focusing on intervention research for five years, Smoke-Free Families opened a National Dissemination Office to promote the widespread implementation of prenatal tobacco treatment across the country. Directed by Cathy Melvin, the National Dissemination Office funded three statewide demonstration projects. The purpose was to test promising approaches for incorporating the 5 A's into clinical practice. The products and lessons learned from these demonstrations would assist other organizations in developing and strengthening their own office systems for treating tobacco dependence.

The three demonstration projects in Oregon, Maine, and Oklahoma used different methods to engage providers in helping pregnant women break their nicotine addiction. In Oregon, the health department focused its efforts on the maternity case management system, in which trained health professionals provide psychosocial support to women in their homes. Protocols for delivering and documenting the 5 A's were used in eight counties and eventually spread to all of Oregon's thirty-four counties. Some of the successful systems changes that were put into place included standardized documentation for tobacco screening and treatment, mandatory cessation counseling training for all new maternity case managers, and new administrative rules that tie delivery of the 5 A's to Medicaid reimbursement.

In Maine, staff members from the demonstration project recruited physician practices from MaineHealth to participate in a nine-month program in which ob/gyns, family practitioners, and midwives attended three face-to-face learning sessions. These sessions were designed to help doctors, midwives, and nurses learn how to incorporate the 5 A's and other techniques into their practices. These methods included a fax referral process to the state quitline and a tobacco treatment database that allowed them to monitor their performance in delivering the 5 A's.

Oklahoma's initiative, Smoke-Free Beginnings, worked closely with Oklahoma State University to encourage compliance with tobacco treatment guidelines. The project succeeded in recruiting twenty-six clinics and practices—ranging from small family medicine offices such as Zachary Bechtol's to an Oklahoma State University clinic with several thousand obstetric patients a year—to enhance their counseling, documentation, and referral process. One unique aspect of the project was the inclusion of healthcare settings that serve American Indians, a population with the highest rates of smoking overall and during pregnancy.[15]

Smoke-Free Beginnings used a unique messenger to propagate its mission: practice enhancement assistants (PEAs) who are nurses or social workers employed by the Oklahoma Physicians Research/Resource Network. The PEA concept, imported from Australia and Europe, is relatively new in America; providers involved in Smoke-Free Beginnings believe that the PEAs were essential to the program's effectiveness. Program staff members also felt that the program gained grassroots popularity among physicians due to its sponsorship by the Oklahoma State Medical Association.

The PEAs' job was not only to coach nurses and doctors how to counsel pregnant smokers, but also to make the entire process an unobtrusive yet essential part of the physicians' practices. Sarah Jane Carlson, who had just received her master's degree in health care business administration, was the project coordinator.

When Carlson and Joy Leuthard, the principal investigator for Smoke-Free Beginnings, launched the initiative, not one of the twenty-six clinics was using the 5 A's to intervene with pregnant tobacco users. Women were typically asked about their smoking status and were advised to quit. But minimal attention was paid to assessing readiness to quit, assisting with a concrete quit plan, and arranging follow-up discussions.

Carlson and her PEAs, who generally worked with each clinic or practice for a year, experienced some resistance at first.

"The doctors have to feel that it's going to work," recalled Carlson. "They did not want to waste their time and waste their breath . . . We thought these practitioners would get on board very quickly. We were very naïve. Some doctors said you would not be able to stop people from smoking. There were a lot of nurses who smoked. But we met with the physician leadership of the practices and explained, 'Here's how to do this. Here's how it works.' One of the great things about pregnant women is that you knew you would see them again and again, and we stressed that you have to move the patients along in the stages of change."

The PEAs visited the clinics every week, making sure that the vividly colored flow sheets were being used in patient charts and that doctors and nurses were documenting their work as they attempted to wean pregnant smokers from tobacco. One of the PEAs, Katy Duncan Smith, stressed this theme: "What's important is to address smoking at every single OB visit. You don't have to take a lot of time, but what's important is to discuss it every time."

The job of Smoke-Free Beginnings was made easier because all the practices belonged to the state's Physicians Research/Resource Network and were, by definition, interested in incorporating new treatments into their practices. Dr. James Mold, who oversees the network in his capacity as director of the Research Division at the University of Oklahoma's Department of Family and Preventive Medicine, said members of the network realized that physicians were increasingly expected to deliver preventive care, rather than just deal with acute crises. "More than 50 percent of premature deaths occur because of four behaviors—sedentary lifestyle, obesity, smoking, and alcohol," Mold said. "Addressing these behaviors ought to be a part of every patient visit. With Smoke-Free Beginnings we tried to systematize the approach to smoking and pregnancy."

Pressures of time and money in the age of managed care, Mold added, make it challenging to move practices in the right direction. "It is remarkably difficult to get practices to change," he said. "You need to understand that primary care practices have no margin. They have no extra energy. They are right on the edge of making it."

A year after the demonstration project ended, neither Carlson nor Mold was certain how well the lessons from Smoke-Free Beginnings had stuck in the twenty-six clinics and practices. But visits to several doctors' offices and clinics showed that the program had become part of the practices' DNA. Although some doctors could not remember all the 5 A's, they did remember 2 A's and an R: Ask, Advise, and Refer. This was true at the University of Oklahoma's Family Medicine Center in Tulsa, which treats thousands of patients a year, many of them uninsured. The center has moved to a system of electronic medical records, and Smoke-Free Beginnings worked with the center's administrators to ensure that questions about smoking—and referrals to quitlines or counseling—are part of the electronically prompted dialogue between doctor or nurse and patient. When they carry their laptops into examining rooms to meet with pregnant patients, physicians and nurses must scroll through a sequence of questions about smoking. "It's a simple way to approach smokers in a systematic fashion," said Brian Lewis, thirty-one, a family practitioner in Tulsa. "You ask all the questions on the screen and you work toward getting them to quit and you address it every visit."

At the Oklahoma Community Health Services clinic—a large center in Oklahoma City that treats mainly Medicaid, Medicare, and uninsured patients—Dr. Suben Naidu, the medical director, has incorporated the techniques of Smoke-Free Beginnings into the clinic's protocols. One of the most enthusiastic converts is Maria Agnes E. Smith, a tall, elegant Nigerian-born nurse-practitioner. Opening piles of patients' charts on her desk, she pointed to the mustard-colored flow sheets, which documented her efforts to persuade pregnant smokers to quit.

"That's my number one issue—right on top," said Smith. "That paper is a reminder. I had a pregnant patient today. She smokes and her partner smokes. She walked in and I said, 'OK, let's talk about smoking.' I could smell the smoke in the air when they walked in. She said she's cutting back. I said, 'How can I help you? You are such a young child and now you are having a child. How can we stop this thing? What can we do to solve this problem?' I told them to quit as a team in expectation of this new person coming into their lives. I think they realized I am on their side. I am not there to knock them."

Institutionalizing Change

The year 2000 was a particularly significant one for tobacco-cessation advocates. That year, the American College of Obstetricians and Gynecologists (ACOG) issued a detailed educational bulletin explaining the 5 A's and their use for pregnant women, and the U.S. Public Health Service released its Clinical Practice Guideline, "Treating Tobacco Use and Dependence," which recommended the adoption of the 5 A's. With the publication of these two bulletins, the medical establishment took a major step toward institutionalizing evidence-based counseling for pregnant smokers. "It wasn't until the guidelines came out in 2000 that there was a real push for translation into practice," Barker recalled. "Those guidelines put the 5 A's into play. And the National Partnership to Help Pregnant Smokers Quit was really successful in bringing all these groups together to endorse and spread this best practice."

The issuance of the federal guideline and the increasingly close relationship between Smoke-Free Families and a newly formed steering committee of seven organizations, including ACOG, led to the establishment, in May 2001, of the National Partnership to Help Pregnant Smokers Quit, a coalition working to promote the use of the 5 A's in prenatal care throughout the country.[16] The partnership currently consists of nearly sixty organizations and agencies such as ACOG, the National Cancer Institute, the Centers for Disease Control and Prevention, the March of Dimes, the American Academy of Pediatrics, and the New York City and North Dakota departments of health. It has dedicated itself not only to spreading the gospel of the 5 A's but also to other proven interventions to help pregnant women quit, such as developing and disseminating evidence-based, pregnancy-specific quitline protocols, working to expand coverage of smoking cessation by Medicaid and private insurers, providing assistance to communities and worksites as they explore ways to help pregnant women quit smoking and provide smoke-free environments, and encouraging continued research into interventions that help pregnant women quit smoking.

The Policy Working Group of the National Partnership worked with five states over the course of a year to either obtain reimbursement for smoking cessation counseling for pregnant women or ensure that current reimbursement was not ended. One notable example was in Kentucky, where, in conjunction with the Campaign for Tobacco-Free Kids and the Kentucky Tobacco-Control Program, legislation was passed for a comprehensive smoking cessation benefit for all Medicaid beneficiaries, including pregnant women, and for an increase in the cigarette excise tax. A pilot project is being planned to explore how to best offer and fund the smoking cessation benefit for pregnant Medicaid recipients in Kentucky as well as in Massachusetts.

Also important was the campaign—led by the American Legacy Foundation—to establish a quitline, Great Start, for pregnant smokers wanting to kick their smoking habit. Cathy Melvin cochaired the committee responsible for developing the counseling protocol and associated materials, and the National Partnership helped to publicize the services of the Great Start Quitline across the country. Today, thirty-eight state quitlines use pregnancy-tailored protocols that are modeled on those developed by the Great Start and the Smoke-Free Families programs.

The Perspective in 2007

A "capstone" meeting held in October of 2006 gave participants in the Smoke-Free Families program the chance to come together and assess the state of the field, the program's accomplishments, and where it had fallen short.

"In 2006, most obstetricians and prenatal counselors were addressing this issue," said Michael Fiore. "There's been a sea change in the last decade. It's an uncommon woman today who gets out of her obstetrician's office without hearing about how you have to quit for you and your baby. I think it's really good news that the rate of smoking among pregnant women is less than 20 percent. That is certainly a success story from where we were in the 1950s, 60s, and 70s."

Today, approximately 25 percent of women who smoke quit spontaneously when they learn they are pregnant.[17] (Estimates of spontaneous quit rates range from 11 to 28 percent for publicly insured pregnant smokers, to 40 to 65 percent for privately insured smokers, who are generally more affluent and better educated.[18]) With proper counseling, a further 10 to 15 percent of women also can be helped to overcome their cigarette addiction—a significant improvement over the 3 to 5 percent of women who, without counseling, typically quit as they move through their pregnancies. Even these relatively modest numbers of women who quit smoking have a sizable impact on the health care system. The ill effects that smoking has on fetuses leads to an estimated $220 to $230 million in additional health care costs at birth and $600 million in additional costs after delivery.[19] That works out to $1,142 to $1,358 in additional neonatal and first-year medical costs for every child born to a smoking mother—financial and human costs that could be avoided with successful 5 A's counseling, which costs a mere $24 to $34 per woman to deliver.[20]

As part of its effort to make augmented 5 A's counseling the standard of care for pregnant smokers, the Smoke-Free Families program funded forty-one projects, some of which demonstrated the effectiveness of other therapies, including the use of financial incentives to spur women to quit. The program and its many partners also worked to persuade state Medicaid agencies and private insurers to cover the cost of counseling, as well as drug and nicotine replacement therapies, for pregnant smokers.

Robert Goldenberg, the national program director of Smoke-Free Families, summed up the role of the program: "If you really want to decrease smoking, which we have, you need to attack it in every possible way. If you think of this as a battle or a war, the shells have been coming from every direction. Smoke-Free Families is a thin wedge in this effort, but it is a wedge. Before Smoke-Free Families, there certainly was no coordinated effort to get pregnant women to quit smoking."

That said, Goldenberg acknowledges that Smoke-Free Families failed to find solutions to two intractable problems. The first is the large number of heavily addicted pregnant smokers who never quit smoking, even after 5 A's counseling. And the second is the extremely high number of women—between 60 and 70 percent—who resume smoking within months of delivering their babies.

"What we're left with is a group of women who are particularly difficult to treat," said Goldenberg, who is now professor of obstetrics and gynecology at Drexel University College of Medicine in Philadelphia.

"They are generally poor white women who are heavy smokers. Everyone in their family smokes and they smoke a lot and nobody has had an impact on getting them to quit. They tend to have smaller babies, less healthy babies, and more babies that die. And because they are poor, they tend to have the least amount of resources to take care of the baby."

"The other bad news is that many women have no intention of stopping forever. They know it's bad for the baby, but when they have the baby they often go back to smoking, and we haven't figured out in any way, shape, or form how to prevent this. We are most successful in getting people to stop who are least addicted. That's also a failure in a way because the ones who are most addicted are the ones most at risk in terms of health."

Despite these specific drawbacks, the program, according to Orleans, "tested many promising interventions, educated the field by adding a number of important studies to the literature, and incubated a potentially sustainable new intervention involving the provision of small incentives to pregnant smokers. Perhaps its greatest success, however, was to build critical evidence, and practitioner and policy support, for what is now regarded as the best practice standard for tobacco-cessation intervention in pregnancy—the augmented 5 A's."

The multifront war on smoking has clearly paid off, with smoking rates cut in half over the last fifty years. Smoking among pregnant women also is steadily waning, although one recent trend—the leveling-off of smoking reduction among girls eighteen to twenty-four—is worrisome. "The good news is that we're at the lowest level of smoking in decades," Steven Schroeder said. "The bad news is that there are still four hundred thousand people dying from smoking every year in the United States. Robert Wood Johnson was the first foundation to take on smoking. We put a lot of research into the field. We're part of that success story. Frankly, we've made more progress than I thought we'd make. But we shouldn't pat ourselves on the back. The tobacco industry is still spending $13 billion a year on marketing in the U.S."

Orleans is similarly cautious about Smoke-Free Families and other tobacco control programs. "Only 3 percent of the $246 billion set aside in the landmark 1998 settlement with America's tobacco companies was actually used for tobacco cessation and control," she said. "There is too little money to advertise an extremely helpful tool—quitlines—and to push for universal coverage by Medicaid and private insurers for cessation counseling. This is shameful."

In the realm of helping pregnant smokers, much remains to be done. This includes funding research into how best to treat heavy smokers who do not quit during pregnancy; how to reach the even larger numbers who jettison the cigarette habit, only to resume smoking after childbirth; and how public policies can be employed more effectively to reduce smoking among pregnant women.

Those involved with Smoke-Free Families are heartened, however, that they have come this far. "Clearly, smoking in general and smoking during pregnancy are a lot less prevalent now than fifteen years ago," Goldenberg said. "There is not a woman in the U.S. who does not know that smoking during pregnancy is bad for her baby and bad for her. That message is clearly out there."

Notes

1. Fiore, M. C., and others. Treating Tobacco Use and Dependence. Clinical Practice Guideline. Rockville, M.D.: U.S. Department of Health and Human Services. Public Health Service, June 2000.
2. U.S. Department of Health and Human Services. Women and Smoking: A Report of the Surgeon General, 2001. (http://www.surgeongeneral.gov/library/womenandtobacco/)
3. Centers for Disease Control and Prevention. "Annual Smoking-Attributable Mortality, Years of Life Lost, and Productivity Losses—United States, 1997–2001." *Morbidity and Mortality Weekly Report,* 2005, 54, 625–8.
4. U.S. Department of Health and Human Services. The Health Benefits of Smoking Cessation: A Report of the Surgeon General, 1990. Rockville, Md.: Public Health Service, Centers for Disease Control, Office on Smoking and Health, 1990. (DHHS Publication No. [CDC] 908416.).
5. Cnattingius, S. "The Epidemiology of Smoking During Pregnancy: Smoking Prevalence, Maternal Characteristics, and Pregnancy Outcomes." *Nicotine & Tobacco Research,* 2004, *6*(Suppl. 2), S125–S140.

6. Orleans, C. T., and others. "Helping Pregnant Smokers Quit: Meeting the Challenge in the Next Decade." *Tobacco Control,* 2004, *9*(3), 6–11.
7. Kluger, R. *Ashes to Ashes: America's Hundred-Year Cigarette War, the Public Health, and the Unabashed Triumph of Philip Morris.* New York: Knopf, 1996.
8. Cnattingius, S. "The Epidemiology of Smoking During Pregnancy: Smoking Prevalence, Maternal Characteristic, and Pregnancy Outcomes." *Nicotine & Tobacco Research,* 2004, *6*(Suppl. 2), S125–S140.
9. Ibid.
10. Centers for Disease Control and Prevention. Behavioral Risk Factor Surveillance System: 2000 Survey Data. (www.cdc.gov/brfss/ti-surveydata2000.htm)
11. Orleans, C. T., and others. "Helping Pregnant Smokers Quit: Meeting the Challenge in the Next Decade." *Tobacco Control,* 2004, *9*(3), 6–11.
12. Donatelle, R. J., and others. "Randomized Control Trial Using Social Support and Financial Incentives for High-risk Pregnant Smokers: Significant Other Supporter Program." *Tobacco Control,* 2004, *9*(Suppl. 3), 67–69.
13. Ershoff, D. H.; Ashford, T. H.; and Goldenberg, R. L. "Pregnancy and Smoking: An Overview." *Nicotine & Tobacco Research, 6*(Suppl. 2), 101–105.
14. Benowitz, N. L., and Dempsey, D. A. "Pharmacotherapy for Smoking Cessation During Pregnancy." *Nicotine & Tobacco Research,* Apr. 2, 2004, *6*(2, Suppl. 2), S189–S202.
15. Centers for Disease Control and Prevention. "Cigarette Smoking Among Adults—United States, 2004," *Morbidity and Mortality Weekly Report,* 2005, *54,* 1121–1124.
16. The partners included the Association of Maternal and Child Health Programs, the Health Resources and Services Administration, the American Association of Health Plans, the Agency for Healthcare Research and Quality, the Centers for Disease Control and Prevention, and the Robert Wood Johnson Foundation.
17. Orleans C. T., and others. "Helping Pregnant Smokers Quit: Meeting the Challenge in the Next Decade." *Tobacco Control,* 2000, *9*(Suppl. 3), 6–11.
18. Melvin, C. L., and Gaffney, C. A. "Treating Nicotine Use and Dependence of Pregnant and Parenting Smokers: An Update." *Nicotine & Tobacco Research,* 2004, *6*(Suppl. 2), 108–124.
19. Adams, K. E., "What Do We Know About Cost-Effectiveness of Smoking Interventions?" Smoke-Free Families Capstone Meeting, October 18–19, 2006. Washington, D.C. PowerPoint presentation available at www.smokefreefamilies.org.
20. Ibid.

CHAPTER 5

The Community Mental Health and Substance Abuse Partnership of Larimer County, Colorado

Paul Brodeur

Editors' Introduction

It is ironic that the most vulnerable members of American society face the difficult, sometimes nearly impossible, task of dealing with multiple systems. People who are homeless, disabled, poor, or recently released from prison—among others—may have to contend with the acute medical care system, the disability system, various social service agencies, and, in some cases, the criminal justice system. One study by two Brown University researchers found that there were 127 agencies serving the disabled in the medium-sized community of Springfield, Massachusetts.[1] The fragmentation of services is a particularly severe problem for people with both mental illnesses and addiction to drugs or alcohol, who are often shuttled between mental health and substance abuse systems, receiving satisfactory services from neither.

In this chapter, Paul Brodeur, an award-winning journalist and former staff writer for the *New Yorker,* discusses an approach to organizing services for people with both substance abuse addiction and mental illness. The large number of people who suffer from co-occurring mental illness and substance addiction is not widely appreciated, even though it affects about 3 percent of the adult population of the United States.[2] Looked at from a different perspective, approximately half of the people with severe mental illnesses also have a substance abuse problem.[3] Individuals with an existing mental illness consume roughly 38 percent of all alcohol, 44 percent of all cocaine, and 40 percent of all cigarettes in the United States, and those who have *ever* experienced a mental illness consume about 69 percent of all the alcohol, 84 percent of all the cocaine, and 68 percent of all cigarettes.[4]

Developed under a grant from the Local Initiative Funding Partners program, a collaboration between the Robert Wood Johnson Foundation and local foundations to support innovative and worthy local projects, the Community Mental Health and Substance Abuse Partnership of Larimer County, Colorado, has established a coalition of public agencies and private organizations to coordinate services for people with these co-occurring conditions.

Repairing the fragmented system of delivering health care services has been a longstanding concern of the Robert Wood Johnson Foundation. The On Loc and PACE (Program of All-Inclusive Care for the Elderly) initiatives integrated acute and long-term care for frail elders by providing social and medical services in an adult day care setting.[5] The Community Partnerships for Older Adults program was designed to coordinate long-term care and social services for elderly people. In the mental health arena, the Mental Health Services Program for Youth and the Program on Chronic Mental Illness both attempted to develop ways to coordinate mental health services in the community.[6] [7]

Notes

1. Allen, S. M., and Mor, V. "Unmet Need in the Community: The Springfield Study." *To Improve Health and Health Care 1997: The Robert Wood Johnson Foundation Anthology.* San Francisco: Jossey-Bass, 1997.
2. Department of Health and Human Services. Mental Health: A Report of the Surgeon General, 1999. (http://mentalhealth.samhsa.gov/features/surgeongeneralreport/home.asp)
3. National Alliance on Mental Illness. "Dual Diagnosis and Integrated Treatment of Mental Illness and Substance Abuse Disorder." (http://www.nami.org/Template.cfm?Section=By_Illness&Template=/TaggedPage/TaggedPageDisplay.cfm&TPLID=54&ContentID=23049)

4. National Bureau of Economic Research. Mental Illness and Substance Abuse. (http://www.nber.org/digest/apr02/w8699.html)
5. Alper, J., and Gibson, R. "Integrating Acute and Long Term Care for the Elderly." *To Improve Health and Health Care 2001: The Robert Wood Johnson Foundation Anthology.* San Francisco: Jossey-Bass, 2001.
6. Saxe, L., and Cross, T. P. "The Mental Health Program Services for Youth." *To Improve Health and Health Care 1998–1999: The Robert Wood Johnson Foundation Anthology.* San Francisco: Jossey-Bass, 2000.
7. Goldman, H. H. "The Program on Chronic Mental Illness." *To Improve Health and Health Care 2000: The Robert Wood Johnson Foundation Anthology.* San Francisco: Jossey-Bass, 2000.

With more than 250,000 residents, including 24,000 students at Colorado State University, Larimer County is one of the four most populated areas in Colorado. Fort Collins, the county's largest city, with a population of about 118,000, is located about sixty-five miles north of Denver and is home to the university. Mile upon mile of fertile farmlands and grasslands lie in the northern and eastern portions of Larimer County; to the west, ranging from north to south as far as the eye can see, looms the majestic front range of the Rocky Mountains. All in all, a dramatic panorama.

Among the people living in its midst, however, a serious public health problem has been growing over the years—a high rate of mental illness and substance abuse. In 2004, nearly a quarter of the residents of Larimer County reported having been diagnosed with depression, up from 18 percent in 1998. Thirty-six percent of residents with low incomes reported having been diagnosed with depression in 2004, compared with 20 percent in 1998. The use of methamphetamine has posed a critical problem in the county. In 2005, 30 percent of Larimer County residents receiving treatment for substance abuse were treated for methamphetamine as their primary drug of use, compared with 19 percent of substance abuse-treatment recipients residing elsewhere in Colorado.[1]

Services for people who have both mental illnesses and substance abuse disorders are typically fragmented; in most communities across the nation, such people do not usually receive integrated treatment for the two conditions simultaneously. Rather, they receive treatment for only one condition at a time, and if they are fortunate enough to receive treatment for the other condition, it is at a separate location at a different time. This was the case in Larimer County.

Erin Hall, who works for the Health District of Northern Larimer County and is the program manager of the Community Mental Health and Substance Abuse Partnership, describes just how dysfunctional the system had become. "At a meeting that took place in 1999, seven case examples written by agencies providing mental health and/or substance abuse services were distributed to and read by members of our steering committee," she recalled. "To their astonishment and dismay, they realized that four of them had written about the same person. 'I think some of you are describing the same man I have,' one of them said. 'Aren't we talking about the fellow who has family in New Mexico?' another asked. Still another member pointed out, 'This is the guy who wears a tattered brown jacket every day.'"

Hall recounts that the committee members were indeed talking about the same man, and they were shocked to realize that none of them had known he was being cared for by other agencies. "We call him Joe, which is not his real name but one we've given him to protect his privacy," she said. "Since then, we've used Joe's story, along with the stories of others, to build a composite picture of what often happens to people who suffer from mental illness and are also addicted. Joe is a really nice guy once you get to know him, and he has a great sense of humor. As a kid in grade school, he seemed normal and outgoing, but during his teens he became withdrawn, his grades suffered, and he developed what he describes as 'a fire in my brain.' By the age of sixteen, he had begun to smoke marijuana, which calmed him and made him feel better, but he soon entered a cycle in which he medicated himself not only by smoking pot but also by drinking heavily. By his early twenties, he was suffering from major untreated mental illness and addiction, which resulted in his not being able to keep a job or make new friends. By the time he was in his thirties, he was living on the street, unable to get a job, and had few if any friends. At the age of forty-five, he embarked upon a nightmarish two-year ordeal during which he was shuffled from agency to agency with little or no treatment coordination.

"After suffering a mental health crisis, he was taken to the Emergency Department of the Poudre Valley Hospital, here in Fort Collins," Hall continues. "From there, he was sent to the Island Grove Regional Treatment Center, a detoxification agency in Greeley, about thirty miles away, and then back to Fort Collins, to the Hope Counseling Center for outpatient substance abuse counseling. Following another crisis, he was admitted to the Emergency Department of McKee Hospital, in Loveland, seven miles south of Fort Collins, and then shipped back here to Mountain Crest, a psychiatric hospital that treats people with mental illness and substance abuse problems. From there, he was sent to the Colorado State Mental Health Institute, in Pueblo, which is about a hundred and twenty miles south of Denver. Following a stay at the Institute, where they treat serious mental illness, he came back to Fort Collins, to receive treatment at the Larimer County Mental Health Center. However, after committing several crimes—Joe has had charges brought against him for driving under the influence, carrying a concealed weapon, and contempt of court—he found himself in the Larimer County Detention Center, where he received a mental health assessment that resulted in his being sent to the Circle Program, a long-term residential program operated by the State of Colorado for people with serious co-occurring mental illness and substance abuse disorders, which is located in Fort Logan, near Denver. However, after completing the program, he went off his medication, started drinking again, and committed another crime that landed him back in the Larimer County Detention Center. It is estimated that during his two years of shuttling back and forth between different agencies, more than a quarter of a million taxpayer dollars were spent to treat Joe, only to have him wind up in jail."

To reform this unfortunate system, the Community Mental Health and Substance Abuse Partnership was established, with the goal of redesigning and improving the way people with mental illness and addictive disorders are evaluated and treated in Larimer County. Funded in part by the Robert Wood Johnson Foundation's Local Initiative Funding Partners program, the Partnership faces the task of creating an integrated system in which thirty-four organizational providers and many individual providers—among them governmental agencies, nonprofit organizations, hospitals, private practitioners, police officers, school teachers, school counselors, clergy, and mental health advocates—collaborate with one another to improve access to, as well as delivery of, mental health and substance abuse services to an estimated thirty-six thousand residents of the county who are in need of them.

The Program Takes Shape

Early concern about the situation in Larimer County arose in 1995, when Carol Plock, an energetic and purposeful woman then in her late thirties, who had recently become executive director of the Poudre Health Services District in Fort Collins, was called by a man named Jack Ewing. He informed her that there was a mental health crisis in Larimer County, as well as throughout Colorado. Plock had previously heard Ewing on a radio talk program, describing his own battle with mental illness and his frustration over how difficult it was for people like him to get access to appropriate mental health care. As it turned out, he had been a leader in suicide prevention in Colorado for many years, and had been instrumental in creating the governor's task force for suicide prevention, which led to the formation of the Colorado State Office of Suicide Prevention.

"I was fascinated by how eloquent, informed, and passionate he was about the connection between mental illness and suicide," Plock recalled. "So I called him back, and we began meeting to discuss ways in which our community might be able to resolve some of the issues involved. Shortly thereafter, the Poudre Valley Hospital held a session at Colorado State University's computer lab so people interested in improving services for those with mental illness could share information about their concerns and ideas. A year later, Jack and the hospital acted as catalysts in the formation of a coalition of people who either had experienced mental illness or had a family member with mental illness, and which included some midlevel managers of agencies that provide mental health services. The group was concerned that people with mental illness were not getting the level of treatment they needed. The coalition called itself the Larimer County Mental Health Network, and among its members were Jack and me, several therapists in private practice, and representatives from the Larimer County Center for Mental Health, the Health and Human Services Department of Larimer County, and the Mountain Crest Behavioral Health Center, a psychiatric hospital affiliated with the Poudre Valley Hospital."

Plock went on to say that in 1998 the Network sponsored a Mental Health Fair during which mental health providers shared information about their services, and a keynote speaker described what it might take to make significant changes in the delivery of such care in Larimer County. "Following the fair, members of the Network developed a long-term vision and mission statement that called for a coordinated and well-funded continuum of mental health and substance abuse services," she continued. "I can't say enough about the value of their contribution in laying the groundwork for changing the system. By that time, however, all of us had come to realize that real change could not be achieved unless we could involve top leaders in the community in the development of a formal process to bring it about. As a result, I spoke with the board members of the Poudre Health Services District, and, together with Michael Felix—a skilled community health development specialist—took on the job of visiting top leaders in order to gauge their interest and commitment."

The extent to which Plock and her colleagues succeeded can be seen in a memorandum, dated February 8, 1999, which stated that the chief executive officers of the Health District, the Larimer Center for Mental Health, and the Mountain Crest Behavioral Health Center had agreed to become involved in a formal mental health planning process to be called the Communitywide Mental Health and Substance Abuse Planning Project. Between February and August, a plan was developed for assessing the nature and extent of the mental health issues facing the community. A key event in this process took place in August, when eighty people attended an open forum to talk about their experiences with the mental health system and give advice on how to improve it.

During this seven-month period, a thirteen-member steering committee was chosen to discuss information gathered about the scope of the mental health and substance abuse problem in Larimer County, formulate a strategy for dealing with it, and report its findings back to the community. In addition to Carol Plock and Jack Ewing, who represented the Suicide Prevention Coalition of Colorado, its members included representatives of mental health and substance abuse prevention organizations and advocates, law enforcement, the local school district, and therapists in private practice.

The steering committee's search for information culminated in a report entitled "Mental Illness and Substance Abuse in Larimer County," dated February 2001, which revealed some disturbing findings:

- Extrapolating from mental health statistics provided in the 1999 Surgeon General's report on mental illness, it was estimated that more than sixty thousand people in the county were affected by a mental health disorder or by substance abuse. Of those, approximately twenty thousand had significant functional impairment caused by mental illness, and fifteen thousand were seriously impacted by substance addiction.

- Major depression was the number one health burden in the community by a wide margin, outranking cardiovascular disease, cancer, and other illness.
- The rate of suicide in Larimer County mirrored that of Colorado and was almost 40 percent higher than the national average.
- One in four inmates in the County Detention Center was taking psychotropic medication. The number of female inmates had tripled in the previous four years. According to statewide data, 75 percent of these women were in need of treatment for mental illness.
- People with mental illness reported difficulties in finding and paying for appropriate treatment. They also reported a lack of understanding about the nature of mental illness within the court and school systems.
- Both consumers and providers of mental health and substance abuse services reported long waiting lists for outpatient care, prescriptions, and treatment for substance abuse.

Following an extensive process that included 241 interviews, several discussion groups, and a community forum, members of the steering committee identified a number of crucial needs that had to be met to overhaul the mental health and substance abuse system in Larimer County and then recommended its top priorities for initial action:

First, to create an improved and integrated mental health and substance abuse information and referral system, the steering committee recommended that the current therapist referral service be expanded into a more comprehensive program that would create linkages (including electronic links) between the twenty-four-hour response system, the crisis response system, and various mental health and substance abuse treatment centers. In addition, it recommended the establishment of a crisis response subcommittee to create a more efficient and understandable response system with clear protocols and responsibilities for evaluating people with mental illness and/or addiction disorders, and for sending them quickly and directly to an appropriate agency for treatment.

Second, to improve the delivery of mental health and substance abuse services to people who did not qualify for Medicaid, as well as those with low incomes who were uninsured, the committee recommended that a policy subcommittee be formed to develop strategies that would result in increased funding for mental health and substance abuse services to the low-income, non-Medicaid population.

Third, the steering committee recommended the creation of a comprehensive education plan that would lessen the stigma of asking for help in dealing with mental illness and substance abuse among the general population and would educate what it called "gatekeepers"—among them school personnel, law enforcement officers, clergy, judges, and employers—in how to identify the signs and symptoms of mental illness and addiction disorders and to make appropriate referrals for treatment. The education plan would introduce specialized training for primary care physicians interested in improving their ability to treat and refer patients suffering from mental illness and substance use disorders. It would also train mental health and substance abuse professionals to increase their knowledge about current treatment innovations, as well as about local resources and protocols for evaluating and referring patients to appropriate agencies.

Fourth, recognizing the need to create and implement an effective infrastructure that would support their broad plan to change the mental health and substance abuse system in Larimer County, the committee, in December 2000, created a consortium of existing agencies, with headquarters adjacent to the Poudre Health Services District, and with funding to be provided by the Health District and Partnership members and through outside grants.

The consortium was called the Community Mental Health and Substance Abuse Partnership, and among its members—thirty-four organizations and some eighty individuals over time—were top executives from all of the major mental health and substance abuse providers in Larimer County, as well as leading representatives from Colorado State University, consumer advocates, officials of the justice system, law enforcement officers, public school personnel, and other interested parties. The Partnership was staffed by Erin Hall, the project manager; chaired by Cheryl Olson, a highly respected former county commissioner; and overseen by the Health District's executive director, Carol Plock. Under their direction and that of the steering committee, new subcommittees began work on phase two—the development of action plans to deal with the four top priorities that had been identified.

The Partnership Takes Shape

During phase one, members of the steering committee had estimated that $18.6 million a year was being spent by sixteen major agencies that provided the bulk of funding to care for tens of thousands of residents of Larimer County who were suffering from some degree of mental illness and substance abuse. Of the $18.6 million, about $11 million was covered by insurance—private, Medicaid, and Medicare—and by other federal and state funding and self-payers. This left a burden of approximately $7.6 million that had to be generated within Larimer County to care for people who were either uninsured or too poor to pay for treatment. Because local funds for repairing the broken mental health and substance abuse system were already being stretched to the limit, the steering committee—recognizing that multiple interventions would have to be undertaken to make the fundamental changes necessary to achieve its vision—recommended that the community partnership submit a proposal for funding the restructuring program to state and national institutions that might be interested in financing such a project.

In late 2001, Ruth Lytle-Barnaby, the executive director of the Poudre Valley Hospital Foundation, read an announcement seeking nominees for funding from the Robert Wood Johnson Foundation's Local Initiative Funding Partners program.* She called Carol Plock with an offer to nominate the Partnership and to serve as its first funding partner. Plock then wrote a letter on behalf of the Poudre Health Services District to Pauline M. Seitz, director of the Local Initiatives Funding Partners Program, requesting a grant of $340,000 over a four-year period starting in August

* Local Initiative Funding Partners is a program of matching grants that was created in 1987 to support collaborative relationships between the Robert Wood Johnson Foundation and local foundations that finance innovative community-based projects in the area of health and health care. The philosophy guiding the program is that local grant makers interested in addressing local health care problems have a knowledge of their communities that no national foundation can match.

of 2002 to support the implementation phase of the Community Mental Health and Substance Abuse Partnership.

In an accompanying project narrative, Plock told Seitz that the current planning phase should be completed by the middle of 2002 and that the implementation phase would require more financial resources than the Partnership could raise locally at one time. She also informed Seitz of the progress being made by the four subcommittees that had been formed to deal with the top priorities.

On April 17, 2002, Seitz and Paul Nannis, a member of the Local Initiative's national advisory committee, made a site visit to the Community Mental Health and Substance Abuse Partnership. Although they had praise for the Partnership's staff and leadership and the high level of cooperation and commitment among its member agencies and local funding foundations, they felt that the project needed to focus its strategies and determine specific measurable outcomes. As a result, they recommended that the Partnership be awarded a one-year planning grant during which the action plans could be completed and initial interventions begun. Based on this recommendation, the Robert Wood Johnson Foundation awarded the Partnership a planning grant of $72,000, to run from July of 2002 through the end of June of 2003.

The Partnership wasted little time in installing the first of its major system changes. In September of 2002, a program called Connections—a specialized service designed to provide mental health and substance abuse information, referrals to appropriate treatment agencies, and other assistance to people who requested help—was established at the Fort Collins headquarters of the Larimer Center for Mental Health. Connections was a collaborative effort of the Center and the Health District of Northern Larimer County—the new name of the Poudre Health Services District. During the next year, counselors at Connections interviewed and assisted several hundred individuals. Meanwhile, staff members of the Partnership trained 127 school system personnel in how to identify mental illness and substance abuse symptoms among students and how to make appropriate referrals to Connections.

Erin Hall describes what happened when a woman called Connections, desperately seeking help for her adolescent son, Peter (a pseudonym). "The mother had recently found Peter's journal, in which he had written about cutting himself a few days earlier," Hall says. "He had also written that his younger brother had walked in on him just as he was holding a gun to his head. Realizing that a mental health crisis was in the making, the counselor who answered the telephone at Connections told the mother to bring Peter to the Mountain Crest Hospital right away, and proceeded to make sure that Mountain Crest was notified of his imminent arrival. A little while later, the mother called back to say that she and Peter were on their way to the hospital, and to thank the counselor for 'making a big difference today.' Afterward, we learned that in her attempt to find help, the mother had initially called Peter's school and spoken with a counselor there, who had advised her to contact Connections. This is a great example of how our Partnership's integrated referral system functions to provide early intervention and prevent tragedy."

In November, 2002, Plock wrote another letter to Seitz, requesting that the Local Initiative Funding Partners program award a three-year, $290,000 grant to the Partnership that would be combined with $485,000 in local funds to finance the restructuring of the way mental health and substance abuse services were being provided in Larimer County. In an accompanying narrative, Plock informed Seitz about the formation of the Connections program, completion of the action plans for dealing with top priority issues, and the development of a model by the Health District evaluation team that would assess the impact of the Partnership's work. Five months later, after a site visit by members of the Local Initiative and a positive recommendation from the team, the Robert Wood Johnson Foundation awarded a $290,000 Local Initiative grant to start on July 1, 2003, and end on June 30, 2007.

During the first year of the implementation grant, Partnership staff members trained an additional 388 gatekeepers—among them school personnel, early childhood educators, and health and human services staff—and made plans to extend the training to law enforcement officers. Nineteen local agencies that provided mental health and substance abuse services signed memoranda of understanding pledging to cooperate with Connections, which served more than seven thousand clients during the period. At the same time, a major effort was begun to organize the crisis and after-hours response system. A critical turning point in this effort came when the Poudre Valley Hospital committed itself to the establishment of a hospital-based crisis assessment center for people with mental illness and substance abuse problems. In addition, the Partnership worked with twenty organizations to change the way they handled crisis situations, including creating a matrix to be used by all initial entry points—for example, the phone numbers 211 and 911, the police, and ambulance services—so that consistency could be achieved in how individual situations were evaluated and appropriate referrals might be made. Finally, the Partnership secured funding to create and sustain an integrated care project with two local primary care clinics, where mental health and substance abuse professionals would work alongside primary care physicians.

Ann Cope, a mental health specialist at the Connections program in Fort Collins, tells the story of a man in his early thirties whom she calls Jeff. He has been referred to the center by court order for a full mental health evaluation because he has been convicted several times for possession and use of methamphetamines and has been in and out of prison. "The evaluation costs $150, however, and Jeff doesn't have money enough to pay for it," Cope says. "In fact, he's so broke that he's been sleeping on the floors of friends. Jeff has had a rough life and was raised in the foster care system. He suffers from severe anxiety and has panic attacks regularly because he fears that people everywhere are going to hurt him. He has been using meth for several years. And is surrounded by other users, including his girlfriend, his boss, and his coworkers.

Cope goes on to say that Jeff's condition had never been diagnosed properly, and on being arrested for possession and use of methamphetamines he had almost always been sent straight to jail. "In the past, the few mental health specialists who examined him insisted that he become clean and sober before they would treat him for mental illness," she explains. "But how could Jeff kick his drug habit when he had become paranoid to the extent of believing that almost anyone he encountered might do him harm? When he was referred to us, he clearly wanted help, but was exceedingly wary of interacting with anyone, so I enrolled him in our Stepping Stones group, which was established in 2004 to create a nonpunitive and flexible environment for people who are not yet ready to embark on therapy. Jeff started attending Stepping Stones meetings regularly, but then he skipped an appointment I had made for him with a pro bono psychiatrist. Not wanting to give up on him, I enrolled him in a program called Projects for Assistance in Transition from Homelessness, where he received a thorough evaluation and an accurate diagnosis and started on medication."

At this point, Cope declares that under the system that existed before the changes brought about by the Partnership, Jeff would probably have gone untreated and been lost, but because the new system allowed her to go the extra mile with him, he slowly came to trust the people who were trying to help him. "Finally, he felt safe enough to tell us what had happened to him," she continues. "Out of the blue one day, he revealed having been the victim of serious sexual abuse while growing up. As a result, counselors from the Projects for Assistance in Transition from Homelessness helped Jeff receive victims' assistance funding, which allowed him to receive intensive specialized treatment damage caused by the sexual abuse he had undergone.

Cope concludes her account of what has happened to Jeff by observing that, like many people with serious mental illness and addiction disorders, his ordeal has proved to be ongoing. "Not long ago, he was hospitalized for being suicidal, with a plan and means to kill himself," she says. "While in the hospital, he was stabilized on his medications and efforts were made to probe deeper into his condition. At the time, he had not used methamphetamines for nearly a year and had found an apartment. However, he faces legal charges as a result of his past meth use and may still return to prison—a prospect that fills him with despair."

During the second year of the grant—the period from July 1, 2004, to December 31, 2005—the Partnership trained 279 more gatekeepers and made plans to extend training to members of the faith community. Working collaboratively with the Colorado Division of Criminal Justice, the Partnership helped coordinate weeklong crisis intervention training sessions for more than fifty local law enforcement officers, who learned how to interact with mentally ill citizens without resorting to violence and to defuse potentially violent situations. Realizing that local physicians needed help diagnosing and treating mental illness and substance abuse problems, the Health District, the Partnership, and the local safety net primary care clinics established a program called Integrated Care in March 2005. Under this program, mental health professionals began working with primary care physicians at two safety net clinics in Fort Collins—the Salud

Family Health Center and the Family Medicine Center—which serve low-income and uninsured patients, who have the least access to psychiatric help. The clinics share a team of mental health and substance abuse specialists who can provide patients with services or make appointments to receive services at the same time patients are visiting their primary care physicians. This integrated approach not only provides more expertise in a single setting but also enables a primary care physician to bring a psychiatrist or a psychologist into the examining room to talk to a patient, and to consult with the mental health specialist about appropriate medication for the patient. During the first four months, nearly two hundred people were treated for mental illness and addiction disorders at the two clinics.

The most significant change during the second year of the Local Initiative Funding Partners grant was the official opening, on February 2, 2005, of the Crisis Assessment Center adjacent to the Poudre Valley Hospital Emergency Department. There, a trained team from the Mountain Crest Behavioral Healthcare Center—including several psychiatric counselors—was on duty twenty-four hours a day to evaluate patients and, depending on the results, to hold them for further assessment, transfer them to a treatment facility, or place them with an appropriate professional. The new center significantly reduced confusion that had previously existed among police officers, ambulance personnel, and others about whether to take a person in crisis to the Emergency Room at the Poudre Valley Hospital, the Mountain Crest Behavioral Healthcare Center, a detoxification facility, or elsewhere.

Thanks to funding provided by several members of the Partnership, patients in need of detoxification could henceforth be transported from the Crisis Assessment Center to the Island Grove Regional Treatment Center, in Greeley, twenty-four hours a day; previously such transportation had been funded for only one shift for five days a week. Moreover, staff members at the Crisis Assessment Center could now make same-day or next-day appointments (not just referrals) for patients with key providers, such as Connections and the Larimer Center for Mental Health. The Partnership also announced that it was developing a system in which private therapists would provide, on a volunteer rotating basis, outpatient appointments if they were deemed appropriate by the Crisis Assessment Center's staff.

A visit to the Crisis Assessment Center adjacent to the Poudre Valley Hospital Emergency Department includes a conversation with Officer L. H. "Bud" Bredehoft, a strapping mustachioed veteran of the Fort Collins police department, who has been stationed for the past several years at the department's downtown substation. Bredehoft is a pioneer in the new way police officers are being trained to deal with people who are mentally ill or exhibit signs of chronic addiction to alcohol or other substances. "For many years, one of our chief concerns at the downtown station has been how to resolve problems posed by the city's homeless population," he says. "In the old days before the Partnership came into being, there was a 'revolving door' in which homeless street people arrested for disorderly conduct or other offenses were sent to the county jail. Clearly, however, the root causes of chronic homelessness are mental illness, substance abuse, or a combination of the two, so a solution to the problem is going to be achieved not through the criminal justice system but by restructuring the way people with mental illness or substance abuse problems are processed. Thanks to the efforts of the Partnership, a police officer can now bring people he deems to be in crisis here to the Crisis Assessment Center, knowing that they will be evaluated and referred to agencies capable of treating them quickly and humanely. This not only benefits the person in crisis but also allows the officer to return to duty much sooner than before."

At this point, Bredehoft describes the weeklong training that police officers in Fort Collins and elsewhere in Colorado are being given to de-escalate tensions and minimize the possibility of physical confrontation when they encounter people suffering from mental illness or the effects of addiction disorder. "Great emphasis is placed upon negotiation in order to achieve an outcome that is in the best interest of the person the officer is interviewing," he explains. "The training, which is extremely realistic, involves intensive sessions in which officers interact with actors playing the role of people who are in the throes of a mental crisis or are under the influence of alcohol or drugs. In this way, police officers are being taught to become advocates for such people, and to consider their well-being." Bredehoft pauses and gives a rueful smile. "Not so long ago, my colleagues at the station were razzing me for being exactly that—an advocate for the homeless."

In the annual report to the Local Initiative Funding Partners program for the final year of the grant, Erin Hall noted that the Partnership had trained 200 more gatekeepers, bringing the total to 1,543, and that it was about to pilot test an educational campaign targeting men with untreated depression among employees of the City of Fort Collins. She went on to say that more than thirteen thousand people had received counseling and assistance at Connections since it was established in September of 2002, and that nearly 4,500 mental health and substance abuse evaluations had been performed by members of the crisis assessment team since the Crisis Assessment Center opened in February of 2005. In addition, mental health and substance abuse specialists working with primary care physicians at the two safety net clinics had treated more than eight hundred patients since the Integrated Care program had begun in March of 2005. Many of these patients were homeless or had recently been released from jail, or were living on low incomes.

Integrating Mental Health and Substance Abuse Services

By mid-2006, the Partnership had brought about many systems changes in identifying people with potential mental illness, substance abuse disorders, or both, by intervening early and effectively and connecting them to help. One of the most difficult problems to address is how to improve the delivery of help for people who have the most severe and complex needs, especially those with co-occurring mental illness and addiction disorders, and who may also confront varying combinations of homelessness, criminal justice problems, and physical disabilities. Helping individuals with such needs will necessitate major changes in treatment, support services, and both transitional and permanent housing.

This ambitious undertaking represents the greatest challenge of all in the attempt to overhaul the mental health system of Larimer County, and it will require considerably more time to become a reality. In the spring of 2005, the Partnership, in collaboration with the Health District of

Northern Larimer County, submitted a proposal for funding that would provide integrated services for people with co-occurring disorders to a project called Advancing Colorado's Mental Health Care—a joint effort of the Caring for Colorado Foundation, the Colorado Trust, the Denver Foundation, and the HealthONE Alliance, which had banded together to finance up to ten five-year projects to help communities improve the integration and coordination of mental health services. In August of 2005 the Partnership and the Health District were notified that they had been selected to receive a five-year, $590,000 grant to carry out the project.

Using money from this grant—together with funding of their own, extension dollars provided by the Local Initiative Funding Partners program, and money from local individuals, corporations, and foundations—the Partnership is embarking on two major projects designed to assist individuals with complex needs in reclaiming healthy lives. The first project is the development of combined services centers—one in Larimer County and other in neighboring Weld County—which would include 24/7 treatment for acute mental illness and detoxification and would create new emphasis on making sure that people with co-occurring disorders receive appropriate treatment. The Weld County combined services center is scheduled to open in late 2007, and it is expected that the Larimer County center will become a reality in 2008.

The second project is the development of an evidence-based model for treating people with co-occurring severe mental illness and substance abuse disorders—a model called *integrated dual disorders treatment.* The new protocol includes changes in treatment approaches, provision of consistent support, assistance in securing specialized employment, and assured housing. In 2006, several Partnership members traveled to Ohio and Illinois to learn about integrated dual disorders treatment, and in early 2007 key partners made the commitment to restructure their services so that the integrated dual disorders treatment model can be integrated locally. Because the model is staff-intensive, it will take a few years for local agencies to complete their restructuring. In the meantime, the Partnership will apply for a grant from the federal Substance Abuse and Mental Health Services Administration to help fund staffing during the phase-in period.

Although these two projects are major, they alone will not be sufficient to transform the system so that it will be able to provide adequate care for people with complex needs. For this reason, the Partnership has begun a reassessment of what has changed since its inception and what changes need to be made in the future. Findings from the reassessment will be used to determine priorities for the next five years.

The Difference It Can Make

Carol Plock assesses the Community Mental Health and Substance Abuse Partnership in terms of whether she and her colleagues have succeeded in creating a system that may provide an entirely different outcome for Joe, whom we met earlier, and for thousands like him. She presents a scenario of what life would be like for people with mental illness and addiction disorders in a system in which they are treated in an integrated manner.

"First of all, imagine a system in which one of Joe's teachers in elementary school realizes that he may be exhibiting signs and symptoms of mental illness," Plock says. "The teacher discusses the matter with the school counselor, and together they arrange a conference with Joe's single mother, who has been concerned about changes in Joe's recent behavior, but delayed seeking help because of concern that she couldn't afford it. The counselor then provides her with the phone number of Connections, where professional staff members find a pro bono psychiatrist and a pro bono therapist to diagnose Joe's problems.

"During an evaluation process," Plock continues, "it is determined that Joe suffers from bipolar disorder. At that point, Joe is given prescriptions for several medications—he has to try three before finding one that provides relief—and his mother receives help in paying for them from the prescription assistance program. Meanwhile, she and Joe work with the pro bono therapist to learn about his disease and to develop ways of lessening its impact on him. In addition, Joe and his mother decide to tell his teacher and the school counselor about the diagnosis so that they can help him manage the disease. Joe's health improves rapidly as a result of his medication and the support of his teachers, and he goes on to complete high school with flying colors. He then enters State University, starts a relationship with a girl he meets there, and decides that things are going so well for him he can do without his medication. At about this time, he falls in with some classmates who don't know that he has a bipolar disorder, and they invite him to drink and smoke marijuana. Almost without noticing it, Joe proceeds to slip into a heavy dependence on illegal substances. Then, after a night of heavy drinking, he tells his girlfriend that he's in despair and has bought a gun so he can end his life."

Plock goes on to say that when Joe's girlfriend fails to persuade him to seek help, she calls 911. "The police officer who responds has received crisis intervention training and, after talking to Joe at length, convinces him that he should go to the Crisis Assessment Center at Poudre Valley Hospital. After asking Joe's permission to access his medical records, the crisis assessment team learns that he suffers from bipolar disease. Because he is still intoxicated, however, they send him to the Combined Services Center, which is equipped to help him through detoxification, as well as help him deal with his mental health crisis. Joe stays at the Combined Services Center long enough for the staff members to get a complete picture of his background and current situation and to counsel him on how to turn his life around.

"Fortunately, because of his former experience with the new mental health system, he takes their advice seriously and agrees to undergo treatment specifically designed for people suffering from co-occurring mental illness and substance abuse disorders. As a result, he goes back on medication for his bipolar disease, finishes college, finds a good job, and marries his girlfriend.

"Our new Joe doesn't have to enter the Integrated Dual Disorders Program—high-intensity treatment that also exists in Larimer County—because knowledgeable people have intervened early enough to get him the help he needed. Nor, unlike the Joe of our earlier story, has he been recycled in and out of multiple agencies without appropriate treatment, only to end up in jail."

Plock concludes her assessment of how Joe might fare in the new mental health and substance abuse system that has been established in Larimer County by acknowledging that only time will tell whether the outcome she envisions will prove to be a reality. "One thing I can say for sure," she says. "The Partnership has improved the system tremendously, and its members intend to keep improving the system until our goals are reached."

Conclusion

The effectiveness of the Community Mental Health and Substance Abuse Partnership of Larimer County and the results it has achieved in a short period are largely due to the remarkable good will and camaraderie of the providers, consumers, advocates, and others that make up its membership. It is to be hoped that attempts to emulate this project will be undertaken in other communities in the nation, where the growing incidence of untreated mental illness and addiction disorders threatens to weaken the social fabric. It remains to be seen, however, whether the unselfish cooperation that exists among members of the Partnership can be achieved in larger venues, or whether such an extraordinary degree of collaboration can best be attained in smaller closer-knit communities, where people may not only tend to be more familiar with one another but also more civic-minded.

Note

1. Compass of Larimer County. Substance Abuse Treatment—Colorado and Larimer County, 2005. (www.larimer.org/compass/substance_abuse_treatment_h_atod.htm#book1a)

CHAPTER 6

The Active Living Programs

Susan McGrath

Editors' Introduction

The built environment—that is, the physical and social environment in which people live—has become inhospitable to physical activity. Towns are built without sidewalks; suburbs are developed with stores reachable only by car; cities lack parks and recreation areas. People no longer walk to work, or to school, or even down the street to talk with their neighbors. Partly as a consequence of sedentary lifestyles, obesity rates have climbed dramatically over the last half-century, leading to increases in diabetes, heart attacks, and other illnesses. Unless something is done to get Americans moving again, their health will continue to decline.

In 2000 and 2001, the Foundation developed a series of Active Living programs designed to restructure the built environment in ways that would make it easier for people to take walks, go for bike rides, or otherwise get some physical exercise. The idea was not a new one, and it had been fashionable in urban planning circles for many years. What *was* new was that a foundation dedicated to improving *health* would seize upon an idea that was basically an urban planning one. Developing and overseeing programs required Foundation staff members—most of whom were trained in the medical care system, public health, or social science research—to expand their horizons and learn about behavioral psychology, urban planning, education, and transportation.

Recently, the Foundation announced a $500 million programming effort to reverse the epidemic of childhood obesity. The lessons from the Active Living portfolio of grants are being applied in the development of programs addressing the issue.

Susan McGrath, the author of this chapter, is a Seattle-based freelance writer specializing in the environment and natural history. Her articles have appeared in *Audubon, National Geographic, Smithsonian,* and other magazines. Prior to becoming a freelance writer, McGrath was an environmental columnist for *The Seattle Times.*

When Howard Frumkin of the Centers for Disease Control and Prevention puts together a PowerPoint presentation on health and the built environment, he likes to disarm his audience with some choice photographs illustrating the lighter side of his subject. The picture he sometimes includes of a man walking his dog out the window of his car is a good one. So is the picture of an escalator connecting the floors of an open-plan, two-story gym. And the couple getting married at a drive-through tunnel of vows in Las Vegas prompts audible chuckles.

But the audience's laughter is rueful. We're a nation of shamefully lazy people, the pictures imply, hopelessly addicted to our automobiles, our escalators, our snow blowers, leaf blowers, and riding lawn mowers. Though we know how critical physical activity is to our health, more than half of us can't manage to fit in even thirty minutes of moderate exercise most days. A quarter of us don't get any regular exercise at all. We move from our beds to our cars to our parking garages to our elevators to our jobs and back again, day after day. Or we simply stay in the house with the television on. We cover so little ground under our own steam that our legs only carry us one and a half miles in a typical week. It's no wonder that coffins come in size triple-wide these days.

Inactivity is epidemic. But its root causes in the United States are far more complex than those pictures suggest. Skillfully, Frumkin begins to build his case. He shows pictures of where we live. First, the outlying areas, where every house sits on an acre or two, each with a road feeding into an artery leading onto a highway—in one case, a twenty-three-lane highway, wider than an aircraft carrier is long. The people who live in these houses will never walk or bicycle to any destination, Frumkin tells us, because they're too far away.

More than half of all Americans live in suburbs these days. The unmistakable "loops and lollipops" of newer suburbs appear on Frumkin's screen. Residents of these paisleyesque cul-de-sacs have to drive half a mile to visit the neighbors on the other side of the fence in their own backyards, he notes. And they can't pick up a gallon of milk at the store without getting in their cars, because not a single shop or business lies within reasonable walking distance of home. They'll have to drive their kids to every play date and play performance, and even to school every day if they're not on a school bus route. Up flash photos of schools in Minnesota and Michigan. Newer schools today are built on cheap land in outlying areas, Frumkin tells us, and are surrounded by acres of asphalt parking lot to accommodate all those buses and cars needed to deliver the students. Fewer than 15 percent of American schoolchildren walked to school in 2003—down from 40 percent in 1970.

But physical barriers to activity aren't endemic to the suburbs. Take a city sidewalk—any sidewalk, Frumkin says. He shows streets with no sidewalks and streets with discontinuous sidewalks; sidewalks that list steeply streetward; narrow sidewalks, broken sidewalks, barren sidewalks; sidewalks perilously close to heavy traffic; sidewalks that lead nowhere; and the pièce de résistance, a sidewalk in the aftermath of a storm. A large tree has fallen across this one, initially blocking both sidewalk and street: the highway crew has come out with admirable speed, sawed the fallen tree off at the curb, cleared the street—and left the sidewalk still barricaded by the trunk.

Long before Frumkin's riff on sidewalks winds to a close, the audience has begun to see the bigger picture. We're not inactive because we're lazy. We're inactive because our environment makes us so. "We've engineered routine physical activity out of our daily lives, and now we have to reengineer it back in," Frumkin says.

That reengineering—and the policy and behavior changes required to sustain it—is the ambitious goal of a relatively new movement in the field of public health called "active living." The active living movement is a long-term, multidisciplinary effort to redesign communities to make routine daily activity—walking to the store, passing up the elevator to take the stairs, riding a bike to work—convenient, safe, pleasant, and popular. A key principle of the active-living movement is that undertaking such a profound, societywide change requires a broad, collaborative approach. Thus, active living unites public health with partners in such diverse fields as transportation, planning, architecture, urban design, public policy, government, and criminal justice.

Although the active-living movement shares some common objectives with other community design initiatives such as Smart Growth (see box), it differs from them in an important if subtle way: improving health is its explicit goal. In 2001, the Robert Wood Johnson Foundation jump-started the active-living movement with grants of $50 million, funding a portfolio of initiatives that came to be known as the Active Living programs.

The view that typical, car-oriented, mid- to late-twentieth-century American cities and suburbs are inimical to the pedestrian—and to quality of life in general—is neither new nor original to the Robert Wood Johnson Foundation. The writer Jane Jacobs was one of the first to fling back the curtain, with the publication, in 1961, of *The Death and Life of Great American Cities*, a brilliant and pitiless attack on "modern, orthodox city planning and rebuilding," three chapters of which address the uses of sidewalks.[1] In recent years, a number of community movements and organizations have formed whose missions include stemming sprawl; preserving open space; reducing environmental damage; increasing density, mixed use, and walkability; and improving public transit. These include movements such as Smart Growth and New Urbanism, which have their roots in architecture, city planning, urban design, and the environmental movement. In addition to these, there is a healthy-communities movement, which seeks to employ a variety of community resources to address health disparities and improve health status and quality of life. To a considerable extent, the active-living movement builds on all of these community movements.

The marriage of public health with planning and design has galvanized the field, infusing it with new resources and energy. Though the Robert Wood Johnson Foundation was an early leader—and is still by far the biggest funder to date—health professionals around the country have become key players in the active-living movement. These include health departments, foundations, the Centers for Disease Control and Prevention (CDC), health insurance companies, and national associations.

A New Way of Thinking About Health

"It grew out of a sense of frustration," says Richard E. Killingsworth, currently the executive director of the Harvest Foundation in Martinsville, Virginia, who had previously served as the director of the Robert Wood Johnson Foundation's Active Living by Design program. In 1997, Killingsworth was a health scientist at the CDC. "We'd been doing all this stuff to promote physical activity—fitness and recreation programs, some changes in physical education policies, 'Go to the gym, go out for a walk'—all the same hoopla we're still seeing surface in the media. And it wasn't working. We were having no effect whatever on the national prevalence. So we knew that we had to move away from the traditional mindset that you have to go to a building, get on a machine, and get your thirty minutes in before you go to work. We needed a whole new paradigm."

In October of 1997, Killingsworth's group at the CDC brought together thirty of the country's top experts in architecture, urban design, city planning, landscape architecture, transportation engineering, community development, and criminal justice, and asked them, "How can we create change that incrementally invites physical activity into the whole day?"

"The consensus was that if we could design a social culture that values physical activity, and an environment that supports it through various policies and programs and its actual physical structure, then we could begin moving the nation in the right direction," Killingsworth says. There was virtually no research on the subject at that time, he says, and no literature from the public health side. There wasn't even a common vocabulary. Nevertheless, a year later, the CDC and some heavyweight partners, including the Federal Highway Administration, the National Highway Traffic Safety Administration, and the National Center for Bicycling & Walking, launched a program—KidsWalk-to-School. It consisted simply of a Web site and a program guide, which was distributed to activist groups nationally. Word of the program spread, and the print run of five thousand guides "flew out the door in a matter of weeks," Killingsworth recalls.

The subject resonated at the Robert Wood Johnson Foundation. Former senior vice president Michael McGinnis, now a senior scholar at the Institute of Medicine, had recently been brought in to the Foundation to develop the health side of its programming, taking up those issues that fall outside the clinic doors, such as behavior, community improvement, and environment. McGinnis shepherded an internal Foundation staff team through a program review to come up with initial priority areas. Interested in the emerging thinking about the problem of inactivity—that efforts to change individual behavior can succeed only if they take place within the context of larger, community-based efforts to remove environmental barriers and promote appropriate social norms—McGinnis and the health staff put physical activity on the short list.

"Inactivity' doesn't have the sinister ring to it that 'drugs' and 'alcohol' do," McGinnis points out. Yet during the 1990s, medical researchers established a powerful connection between physical activity and health.[2] Regular physical activity was found to reduce the risks of heart disease, diabetes, high blood pressure, colon cancer, osteoarthritis, depression, and anxiety. Inactivity was shown to increase those chronic health risks. Sedentary adults were nearly twice as likely as active adults to develop coronary heart disease, for example, and a full third of deaths from coronary heart disease were attributable to inactivity. Researchers found that lack of exercise and poor diet accounted for approximately 14 percent of all deaths in the United States every year, second only to tobacco use, and more than from alcohol, drugs, firearms, and motor vehicles combined.[3]

To combat these ill effects, the 1996 Surgeon General's report recommended that adults engage in at least thirty minutes of moderate activity on all or most days of the week. Research shows that accumulating these thirty minutes of activity in ten- to fifteen-minute increments over the course of the day is as effective as thirty minutes of sustained exercise done all at once.[4]

In combination with the super-sizing of food portions and increased consumption of soft drinks, this level of inactivity has triggered a dramatic rise in obesity.[5] The Surgeon General's 2001 *Call to Action* found that approximately two out of three adults and one out of five children were considered overweight or obese.[6,7] As is the case with inactivity, the problem is especially evident in some minority groups, as well as among those with lower incomes and less education.

McGinnis felt that the best way for the Foundation to get at obesity was through physical activity. He had long been active in the nutrition area, and he knew there was already a substantial array of players in that arena. Philanthropy is fundamentally best suited as gap filling, McGinnis believes, and the gap was clearly on the physical activity side of the equation. "Inactivity and community design were really wide open at that point," he says. "No one was doing anything. So we made physical activity our leading wedge in the diet-activity dyad."

Kate Kraft and Karen Gerlach, two senior program officers who have since left the Foundation, were the primary architects of the inactivity programs, on a team that included Foundation senior scientist and distinguished fellow Tracy Orleans and then–program assistant Marla Hollander, among others. It was an intellectual and creative exercise in many ways, they recall. The team members visited walkable model communities. They studied active-living programs in Canada and Australia, borrowing language and program ideas. They met with the leading thinkers in public health, experts in nonhealth fields, leaders of community movements, activists, and stakeholders, convening a series of conferences that functioned as intense, interdisciplinary brainstorming sessions. "We spent a lot of time going around explaining to traffic engineers and zoning officials how their decision making affects people's health," Kraft recalls.

The team adopted an approach that would address inactivity at three levels: "upstream," "midstream," and "downstream." Upstream efforts work at the policy level: educating government officials about the health benefits that physical activity confers on their constituents and, indirectly, on government budgets; helping them anticipate and weather opposition from citizens fearful of change in their neighborhoods and from developers resistant to increased regulation and higher building costs; and working to make transportation policies more supportive of physical activity. Midstream efforts act at the community level: establishing programs such as Walking School Bus, for example, and making infrastructure improvements such as bike paths, sidewalks, and gyms. Downstream efforts address the individual level: introducing programs that encourage individuals to adopt healthier lifestyles. The team also looked at private-sector models of social marketing techniques to create consumer demand.

"We didn't set out to design a portfolio of programs," Kraft says. "But when we stepped back from it, we found we had this amazing group of activities all heading in one direction." Kathryn Thomas, a Foundation communications officer new to the team, suggested branding the programs with a single tagline, creating a coordinated identity that told people how the pieces fit together and let each program benefit from the exposure and good work of the others. The team settled on "Active Living."

The Foundation ultimately rolled out a portfolio of six Active Living programs with grants totaling $55 million:

- Active for Life tests evidence-based programs aimed at changing individual behavior in adults age fifty and older.
- Active Living Research supports research into the environmental and policy influences on active living.
- Active Living Resource Center supplies information and technical assistance to communities.
- Active Living Leadership is the policy arm that provides expertise and technical support to government leaders.
- The Active Living Network supplies information and technical assistance to professionals in non-health fields.
- Active Living by Design funds community partnerships that work upstream, midstream, and downstream to make their towns or cities more activity friendly.

Active for Life

Despite the excitement generated by the prospect of launching a broad-based, socioecological approach to inactivity, there was still strong support within the Foundation for more traditional programs aimed at changing individual behavior. As McGinnis explains it, "We knew that taking on a societal behavior change so counter to prevailing public practices as reversing sedentary lifestyles was going to be tough and slow, so, in addition to building toward the broader, long-term change that was necessary—that is, making the built environment more conducive to routine activity—we funded a smaller partner program that promised a nearer-term payoff: a focus on behavior interventions for older people."

Authorized initially in April of 2001, Active for Life: Increasing Physical Activity Levels in Adults Age 50 and Older tests two evidence-based interventions for individual behavior change to see whether they can be expanded and replicated on a national level. "For twenty years, we've seen experimental programs designed to get older people more active," says Marcia Ory, a professor at the School of Rural Public Health at Texas

A&M University and the national program director. "Would their results translate to real-world settings? Our goal with Active for Life was to take the interventions that we knew worked in research settings, apply them to populations that are representative of reality, and see if they could be effective there."

Ory's team spent the first year scrutinizing studies that seemed to hold promise. The group eventually chose two proven interventions: a Stanford University, one-on-one, telephone-based counseling program called Active Choices and a program developed by the Cooper Institute and Human Kinetics, Inc., called Active Living Every Day, which brought participants together in groups for weekly meetings. In January 2003 the Foundation awarded grants to nine organizations at twelve sites.

Early results have been encouraging. A study conducted by Sara Wilcox, an associate professor at the University of South Carolina's Arnold School of Public Health who heads the team evaluating the program, and her colleagues that was published in the *American Journal of Public Health* concluded, "The first year of Active for Life demonstrated that [the] two evidence-based physical activity programs can be successfully translated into community settings with diverse populations."[8] The senior Foundation program officer who oversees the program, Terry Bazzarre, noted, "What's compelling about this work is that it was done in real-world communities with a population that's more difficult to reach and probably much less healthy than the populations in the original studies funded by the National Institutes of Health."

Active Living Research

"Leaders in fields like parks and recreation, city planning, and transportation have a lot of skills for understanding places; in public health and the behavioral sciences we have a lot of skills for understanding people," says James Sallis, who is a professor of psychology at San Diego State University and the director of Active Living Research. "Putting them together," Sallis says, "you're able to understand how people interact with their environment and how you can improve those interactions by improving the environment."

Active Living Research funds investigator-initiated research designed to identify environmental factors and policies that influence physical activity. In five years of operation through April 2007, Active Living Research has funded eighty-five research projects. It also provides its research team members with technical assistance and holds annual conferences where researchers in different areas have a chance to exchange information about methodology and ideas. The program also helps disseminate results, funneling information to policymakers and, through the media, to the public at large.

Investigators come from a wide array of disciplines, representing at least twenty fields. For example, Robert Brown, an assistant professor of criminology at Indiana University-Purdue University, Indianapolis, is looking at how crime and the perception of crime affect people's use of Indianapolis's extensive trail network. "I'm tracking crimes on the trail itself and crimes in the neighborhood of the trail, and that poses a question from the start," Brown says. "How do you define the neighborhood of the trail? Is it within a block? Half a mile? Does it include the parking lot where a trail user parks a car?" Now Brown is turning the tables and looking at the impact of trails on crime, addressing the commonly held perception in the United States that trails are conduits of crime—a perception that trail activists constantly battle.

Kimberly Shinew, an associate professor in the Department of Recreation, Sport, and Tourism at the University of Illinois in Urbana-Champaign, is investigating setting and its impact on physical activity in the Latino population in the Chicago area. One of the settings Shinew studied is a sports facility well attended by Latinos of both sexes. Latino men go there to play soccer, the researcher found, but Latino women go there to watch the men play, getting little or no exercise while at the sports center. Shinew also monitored trail use. "Anglos used the trail in what we consider the traditional way—they go to it and walk for thirty minutes to get their exercise," Shinew reports. "The Latinos used it almost exclusively on a Sunday, and essentially as an open green space, setting up their barbecues beside it, for up to four hours at a time. So there's nobody on the trail, but all these picnic chairs and tents beside the trail." Because the Latino population is growing so fast in some neighborhoods, Shinew says—in some areas going from 5 percent to as much as 40 percent in a decade—these cultural differences have important policy implications for how communities allocate their parks budgets.

At the Department of Design and Environmental Analysis at Cornell University's College of Human Ecology, Nancy Wells, an environmental psychologist, is studying activity levels in people moving to Habitat for Humanity housing in Georgia, Alabama, and Florida, to determine how housing quality affects physical health. Do neotraditional neighborhood design features like small lots, porches, and sidewalks really encourage walking? Do conventional, car-oriented suburban features like loop-and-lollipop street design, big lots, and no sidewalks discourage walking? Might it be worth spending scarce public resources to retrofit suburban neighborhoods to make them more pedestrian friendly? Stay tuned for answers, says Wells, whose results have been submitted for publication.

Active Living Research issued its seventh call for proposals in 2007. Marjorie Gutman, formerly a senior evaluation officer at the Foundation and now a consultant, has been conducting an evaluation of the program. An in-house summary of the survey of grantees and nonfunded applicants concludes that the program has made "rapid progress on the main Active Living Research goals of building an evidence base, building capacity of researchers, leveraging funding, informing policy debates, and providing service to applicants and grantees." Informal conversations with active-living researchers tend to support that conclusion, as does a glance at the professional literature: hundreds of papers on related topics have been published in the past four years.

The Active Living Resource Center

The mission of the Active Living Resource Center is to provide information and technical resources to community and grassroots groups working to encourage walking and bicycling. The resource center is managed and staffed by the National Center for Bicycling & Walking—a nonprofit organization based in Bethesda, Maryland, with a long history of supporting individuals, organizations, and agencies trying to create bicycle-friendly and walkable communities.

The Active Living Resource Center uses its Web site as a portal to connect with communities, placing an emphasis on simple and straightforward language and practical guidance. Its staff members also make "house calls" to needy communities, providing training, outreach, and workshops to help local advocates organize and get programs started, says Bill Wilkinson, the center's executive director. A principal Active Living Resource Center program is Safe Routes to School. Patterned after a program initiated in Denmark in the 1970s that reduced pedestrian and cyclist casualties by 80 percent in ten years and then was expanded to Great Britain and Canada, Safe Routes to School attempts to get children to walk or bike to school and to make routes to school safer. Under Safe Routes to School, communities have, among other activities, organized "walk to school days"; incorporated walking into after-school events; worked with police, crossing guards, and parents to enforce traffic laws; and collaborated in a "walking school bus," in which schoolchildren, accompanied by responsible adults, walk to school in a group. In 2006 the Active Living Resource Center staff began work on City-Safe Routes to School, a variation of the Safe Routes to School program specifically for populations in heavily urbanized environments where schools are typically located in the middle of cities with row homes, multifamily dwellings, and industrial neighbors. In fall of 2006, the Active Living Resource Center held City-Safe Routes to School workshops in Chicago, Birmingham, and St. Paul, Minnesota.

Active Living Network

The Active Living Network serves a function similar to that of the Active Living Resource Center for professionals in the different disciplines collaborating in the active-living movement. "Our objective is to promote collaboration across sectors," says Welling Savo Justin, the director of the Active Living Network, which is based at Pyramid Communications in Seattle. "We serve urban planners, transportation engineers, architects, bike and pedestrian advocates, and professionals in public health and the environment committed to creating active, healthy communities." The network's primary outreach tool is its Web site, where, among other resources, professionals can find narrative descriptions of active-living projects all around the country.

Active Living Leadership

The Foundation had already racked up almost a decade of experience in tobacco control and substance abuse as the health behavior group was formulating a strategy for taking on inactivity. "We'd learned a lot about how to do it and how not to do it," Karen Gerlach says. "One of the big things that rang out to us is that we hadn't enlisted policymakers early on. The Foundation can't lobby, but we certainly can educate leaders such as mayors and state legislators to help them understand how policy change can have an impact." The policy-oriented program that emerged was called Active Living Leadership.

The program, whose National Program Office was originally located at San Diego State University and is now located at the Washington, D.C.–based Global Policy Solutions, started small, getting off the ground in 2002 with three institutional grantees—the National Governors Association, the International City/County Council Management Association, and the Local Government Commission—and a concentrated effort in California, Colorado, Kentucky, Michigan, and Washington. Three additional organizations joined the program in the second year, and the program went national. Today, there are ten grantees: the original three plus the National Association of Counties, the National Conference of State Legislatures, the National League of Cities, the United States Conference of Mayors, the American Association of School Administrators, the Council of State Governments, and the National Association of Latino Elected and Appointed Officials Educational Fund.

"We're working in collaboration," says Larry Morandi, the director of state policy research at the National Conference of State Legislatures. "For instance, the National Conference of State Legislatures, the National Governors Association, and the Local Government Commission looked at the state of Washington and said, 'Here's an opportunity for the three of us to identify stakeholders within our constituencies—governors, legislators, and local government officials—and help them as they consider policy changes.' So in 2004 we held a workshop in Seattle where we brought together state agency directors and legislators and local officials dealing with public health, transportation, and land use, and looked at policy options to try to encourage greater physical activity, access to healthy foods, and so on. The result was legislation introduced in the 2005 session, and when the bill was being heard in committee the Conference of State Legislatures was asked to testify—not to lobby but to talk about how the proposed legislation might meet the legislature's objectives, how it compared with policy approaches being considered in other states. A 'here are your options' kind of thing. And the legislation passed with very substantial margins."

Active Living by Design

Active Living by Design, the hands-on component of the active-living portfolio, funds twenty-five action-oriented, multidisciplinary community partnerships that are developing and implementing local projects that support physical activity and active living. The Active Living National Program Office is based at the School of Public Health at the University of North Carolina at Chapel Hill. Richard E. Killingsworth directed the program from December 2001 through May 2005. Sarah Strunk, a clinical instructor in the school's department of health policy and administration, was the deputy director and took over as director in October of 2005.

Active Living by Design's original call for proposals required applicants to address four strategies:

1. Create and maintain an interdisciplinary partnership that addresses active living.
2. Increase access to and availability of diverse opportunities for active living.
3. Eliminate design and policy barriers that reduce choices for active living.
4. Develop communications programs that create awareness and understanding of the benefits of active living.

The twenty-five community partnerships that ultimately received Active Living by Design grants are a diverse group of entities, as are their settings, which include Honolulu, the South Bronx, the Smoketown neighborhood of Louisville, Albuquerque, five neighborhoods in Seattle, and the college town of Columbia, Missouri. Their tactics vary, too, but most include such efforts as increasing the number of parks, trails, and community gardens; promoting transit and bicycle-commuting possibilities; changing local zoning laws to require sidewalks in new developments and redesigning street standards; developing walking clubs and programs such as Safe Routes to School; encouraging employers to provide bike lockers, showers, and gym memberships for their employees; engaging local elected officials and the media; and raising public awareness about the relationship between inactivity and the built environment.

Active Living by Design takes what Sarah Strunk calls a "high touch/low dollar" approach to grant making. That is, it makes relatively modest financial contributions to the community partnerships—just $200,000 over five years for each site—but provides generous support in the form of high-quality technical assistance to build capacity in the twenty-five demonstration communities.[9] "The program encourages the community partnerships to be creative in seeking additional sources of support and helps them use the Foundation's grant as a launching pad," Strunk explains. "The model is based on the assumption that a modest amount of funding over five years coupled with technical assistance is more replicable and sustainable than a larger, shorter-term grant."

Through the first three years of the program, Strunk says, the community partnerships secured $129 million from other sources to support Active Living initiatives in their project areas, a huge number relative to the Foundation's initial investment of nearly $5 million in grants. The National Program Office has held itself to the same standard. Although the Foundation is still its primary funder, Active Living has brought in four significant grants and contracts, totaling roughly $1.7 million.

How the program's structure and vision play out in the real world is best seen through a look at individual community partnerships. Two profiles are offered here: Bike, Walk, and Wheel: A Way of Life in Columbia, and Active Seattle.

Columbia, Missouri

It's the last Wednesday of the month and Bike, Walk, and Wheel is holding its monthly management team meeting at the kitchen table of its director Ian Thomas. Besides Thomas—who is the director of the community partnership's lead organization, the PedNet Coalition—the team includes Chris Walthall, PedNet's schools program coordinator, and Stacia Reilly, a health educator at the Columbia/Boone County Health Department. Thomas's is a fairly typical suburban house on a wide, curved, suburban street of the type demonized by opponents of sprawl. A hundred yards beyond the kitchen window lies the answer to why a pedestrian advocate might choose to live in a loop-and-lollipop neighborhood: a bucolic gravel rail-trail that runs from downtown Columbia nine miles to the Missouri River.

Thomas, a lanky experimental physicist turned activist, leads the team through the administrative exercise of filling out the previous month's progress reporting system updates. Next item: Passport to Fitness, a year-long, elementary-school-based, physical activity challenge program this community partnership has created and runs, engaging 2,100 kids throughout the school district. How's the new booklet layout coming? Are the prizes offered—a packet of coupons to the local activity and recreation center and roller rink—leaning too heavily on the same businesses? Is their appeal getting stale? The program requires the kids to bring their logs to their physical education teacher to sign; one teacher has asked to keep the booklets at school because so many of her students come from disadvantaged homes where parents may be too overwhelmed to deal with one more task. How can the team make this wrinkle work? Lastly, promotion: the team debates pitching individual PTAs, getting blurbs in school newsletters, on school bulletin boards, and displayed in stores, staging assemblies at school. A daunting action list results.

On to the next items: Walk-to-School Day events, Walk/Bike Safety Education (Walthall gleefully recounts dropping a pumpkin from the stage at school assemblies, then dropping another that is strapped into a bike helmet), and Walking School Bus. The partnership now runs sixteen Walking School Bus routes, each with a dozen or so kids led by two trained adults, to six schools every day. Thomas quotes a boy in his "bus" who announced, "I love the Walking School Bus. It's like recess before school!" When the team turns to promotion—and discussion of every program on this agenda concludes with "better promotion ideas"—Thomas suggests putting the kid's words to use.

Under the agenda item "other business," Thomas updates Walthall and Reilly about a city contract they've applied for. Columbia has been awarded a $25 million non-motorized-transportation pilot project grant from the Federal Highway Administration to help build a citywide bike/walk system. The PedNet Coalition hopes to land the contract to run the promotion and education part of that grant. It is widely expected to get the job, given its track record. In its first year of operation, picking up an ongoing PedNet project, the new partnership led a successful push to adopt new pedestrian-and-bike-friendly citywide street standards—going head to head with developers who absolutely opposed the changes.

"For many years, PedNet was playing this terrible catch-up game," Thomas says. "We'd hear about a new road that was being designed. We'd run around trying to arrange meetings with the public works staff and we'd finally get to see these plans for this new road—well, there's no *sidewalk* there. And there's a housing development here and there's a school there and there's a business district here, so why aren't they putting a sidewalk in so people can actually walk instead of having to use the car all the time? Well, sometimes we were too late and the whole process had moved beyond the stage of being able to add a sidewalk even if we were able to convince them to do it, which was not a given. So that was when we started working on policy.

"The great thing about policy is you can basically save yourself having to run around after every single new road that's being designed. If you can change the policy, then all you have to do is make sure they're following the policy—which is not a given."

PedNet was an all-volunteer grassroots organization with no budget before it formed the community partnership with twenty-nine other organizations and won an Active Living by Design grant. In the first year or two after receiving the grant, Thomas says that he relied heavily on guidance from Rich Bell, his project officer at the National Program Office in Chapel Hill. He feels more comfortable now, but the city contract, if PedNet lands it, would triple the organization's budget, forcing Thomas to hire more staff and move out of his basement and into central offices. Lately, Bell has been helping him find training materials and courses he might take to improve his management skills. "That's the type of thing they encourage us to ask them for," Thomas says. "They're a resource for the twenty-five community partnerships, and they want to help us any way they can."

Thanks to Active Living by Design, the partnership has learned to enlist a broad array of voices in the community and to wield the universal value of public health on behalf of walkability, which otherwise tends to be seen as a luxury item. In the street standards fight, for instance, "We'd phone around to doctors, teachers, and the business owners who were supportive of our position, urging them to go to the planning and zoning meetings. We'd explain why these street standards would be so much better for the health of people, for the kids walking to school who'd do better at their education because they'd had this exercise, for the business owners because a totally car-oriented community isn't good for their businesses, for the disability community and how *desperately* they need sidewalks to get around. We were able to present a very comprehensive argument. And it passed."

Active Seattle

On a rainy early December night at one of Seattle's busiest neighborhood intersections, a chicken is crossing the road—with the "walk" sign, of course, hence this chicken's battle cry of "Wok, wok, wok, walk!" Accompanying the chicken is an assorted group of neighborhood activists carrying signs reading, "Try the view from the crosswalk," "Stop and look," and "Come walk with us!" "This is the heart of the Lake City neighborhood business district," says Erika Berg, a resident inspired to become a pedestrian activist by a few close calls in the crosswalks. "Main Street here is a highway—State Route 522. I've had some scary experiences here, and I've witnessed plenty more."

The group is staging a "crosswalk action," a pedestrian awareness demonstration that makes drivers more aware of crosswalk law and pedestrian safety at dangerous street crossings. Local department of transportation records show at least sixteen incidents involving pedestrians at this intersection in the last three years, says David Levinger, who served as the executive director of the pedestrian awareness organization, Feet First, through April of 2007. It's easy to believe: here are a man in a yellow chicken suit, two leashed dogs, and a dozen men, women, and children—one driving a wheelchair, four carrying large electric-yellow placards, and three wearing Santa caps—marching across the intersection every time the light changes, and cars are turning left through them, past them, and around them as if they weren't even there. "A left turn is the riskiest maneuver drivers make, because it's cognitively so complex," Levinger says. "King County Metro trains its bus drivers to make left turns at five miles per hour. In fact, bus drivers have killed several pedestrians recently while turning left."

Few are the conversations in which Levinger doesn't mention the violent recent death of a pedestrian, and he usually refers to the victim by name. "When Tia was killed," he says. "When Joe was hit." What drives Levinger appears to be a sense of outrage: it's not right that people should have to risk their lives if they choose to walk. But it wasn't until Feet First received an Active Living by Design community partnership grant and became immersed in the values of the Active Living Movement that his sense of outrage got some muscle behind it, he says.

"Feet First had a fairly naïve and unsophisticated rationale for why we were doing what we were," Levinger says. "We certainly had not had health as a central part of our mission. We were more focused on the rights of pedestrians than we were on making a case for why policymakers stand to benefit from improving the environment. Now pedestrian advocacy has become defined with health as a central tenet."

Feet First was a small pedestrian activist group that hadn't quite gotten around to applying for 501(c)(3) nonprofit status when it joined forces with core partners Public Health-Seattle & King County, the Seattle Department of Transportation, and twenty-seven other organizations to respond to the Active Living by Design call for proposals. "That's one of the things about Active Living by Design," Levinger says. "They funded a lot of community partnerships that were small or struggling or had no paid staff. That meant that they ended up with groups that formed themselves around the core values of Active Living by Design, using the Robert Wood Johnson Foundation model and approach. The grants legitimized these small groups. I've seen some of them grow dramatically in this time period—Feet First included—and for me this work has gone from being an avocation to a profession. This is real capacity building."

Active Seattle (the project's overall name) had targeted five Seattle neighborhoods for programs, physical improvements, and promotions to increase walkability. It has landed state grants to implement three Safe Routes to School programs with walking school buses and street improvements, and it leads regular seniors walking groups in its target neighborhoods. The group publishes walking maps of its neighborhoods, showing destinations such as bakeries and bookshops, public bathrooms, and parks. "We're working with doctors in neighborhood clinics to encourage them to address activity with their patients and distribute our maps." A walk-to-shop program in the low- and middle-income Delridge neighborhood will eventually make it possible for residents to check out not only their groceries but also their shopping carts—walking groceries home instead of having to load them into a car and drive or lug heavy bags onto and off the city bus.

Working closely with the mayor's office, Active Seattle successfully advocated for $875,000 in the 2006 budget for sidewalks and stairways—Seattle is a hilly town—and won almost $2 million more from the real estate excise tax for sidewalks and crossing improvements. The community partnership has pushed for changing city policy so that sidewalks will be required of developers building just a few units of housing. "Right now, the city has a threshold of six units," Levinger explains. "But a developer can build an eight-unit complex in two sets of four and sidestep the sidewalk requirement. That's a loophole we're going to change." Every street should have a safe sidewalk along it, Levinger believes. Everyone is a pedestrian.

Conclusion

In the late 1990s, the Robert Wood Johnson Foundation recognized the importance of encouraging people to get more exercise as a way to improve health. Statistics showed that despite two decades of efforts by public health officials and practitioners, people were even less active than they had been when the problem was first identified. Emerging research suggested that no small part of the problem is the built environment—modern urban design and land-use patterns often make routine daily physical activity possible only for a heroic few. Streets are designed to facilitate driving, not walking. Intersections are so wide that, as one activist noted, you need a car just to get across them. Stairwells are hidden away in sterile, airless shafts behind heavy steel fire doors. Sidewalks are *pro forma*. State zoning requirements push new schools far out into the countryside. Older, urban schools are often surrounded by unsafe streets with heavy traffic.

Simply urging people to get more exercise isn't enough to overcome these barriers. A new approach was needed, and the Robert Wood Johnson Foundation took the unusual step for a health foundation of developing partnerships with urban planners, environmentalists, transportation engineers, and landscape designers to launch a series of transdisciplinary programs—the Active Living programs—whose goal was to transform the built environment.

Five years down the road, the former Foundation senior vice president Michael McGinnis says, "The intersecting nature of the domains of influence on health behavior and health outcomes is much more clearly understood now, so there's a greater awareness of the need to tend to the environment if we're going to make a difference. And there is now a growing set of successful efforts about ways in which environmental change might be effected to promote activity."

Though it would be an exaggeration to say the movement is catching fire around the country, as the inactivity and obesity alarm bells grow increasingly clangorous, there is evidence that sparks are flying. "Robert Wood Johnson is still the biggest funder," says the Active Living by Design project officer Richard Bell, "but local and state health departments, public health nonprofits, the CDC, Kaiser Permanente, North Carolina and Minnesota Blue Cross Blue Shield, local hospitals and health-oriented foundations, and a number of national health-related associations have all become significant participants in active living." The response of these organizations is an indication that the movement for creating healthy communities is moving forward.

As the Active Living programs were being designed in the 1990s, obesity had not reached the staggering proportions that it has in 2007. Today, recognizing the great damage that obesity is doing to the nation's health, the Robert Wood Johnson Foundation has made halting, or even reversing, the obesity epidemic among its highest priorities. It is focusing its efforts on children. In April of 2007, the Foundation's president and chief executive officer Risa Lavizzo-Mourey announced a five-year, $500 million effort aimed at addressing childhood obesity.

The focus on childhood obesity has, of course, implications for the Active-Living portfolio, and the Active-Living portfolio offers lessons about how the built environment can be modified to encourage young people to be more physically active. These lessons are informing the development of the Foundation's childhood obesity efforts. Some of the programs, such as Active Living Research, will be continued and refocused on children. Active Living Leadership was renamed Leadership for Healthy Communities in 2004 and its mission expanded to include a focus on healthy eating. In 2005, the Foundation expanded the mandate of Active Living by Design to include healthier eating in twelve of its partnerships. The Foundation's current grant runs through November 2008, and the program's continuation will be considered prior to that date. Active for Life, the Active Living Network, and the Active Living Resource Center will not be renewed, to the great regret of many in the field.

Whatever the Foundation's role in the future, it spawned a movement that is likely to continue. "Active Living is still in its infancy," Richard Killingsworth says. "It will probably take another ten to fifteen years for this stuff to really get off the ground, and two generations of work before we might see real societal change. We need to develop a national agenda about policy and practice and test the things we're implementing. A call to action needs to be made by the Surgeon General or a cabinet official—the Secretary of Health and Human Services or Transportation. This is a very long-range issue. We've started the effort; people are aware of it. But it's going to take decades to play out."

Notes

1. Jacobs, J. *The Death and Life of Great American Cities.* New York: Random House, 1961.
2. U. S. Department of Health and Human Services, Centers for Disease Control. Physical Activity and Health: A Report of the Surgeon General, 1996. (http://www.cdc.gov/nccdphp/sgr/contents.htm)
3. Mokdad, A., and others. "Actual Causes of Death in the United States." *Journal of the American Medical Association,* 2000, *284,* 1238–45.
4. U. S. Department of Health and Human Services, Centers for Disease Control and Prevention. Physical Activity and Health: A Report of the Surgeon General, 1996. (http://www.cdc.gov/nccdphp/sgr/contents.htm)
5. United States Department of Health and Human Services, Public Health Service, Office of the Surgeon General. The Surgeon General's Call to Action to Prevent and Decrease Overweight and Obesity, 2001. (http://www.surgeongeneral.gov/topics/obesity/)
6. U.S. Department of Health and Human Services, National Center for Health Statistics. Prevalence of Overweight and Obesity Among Adults: United States 2003–2004.
7. U.S. Department of Health and Human Services, National Center for Health Statistics, Prevalence of Overweight Among Children and Adolescents 2003–2004. (http://www.cdc.gov/nchs/products/pubs/pubd/hestats/overweight/overwght_child_03.htm)
8. Wilcox, S., and others. "Results of the First Year of Active for Life: Translation of Two Evidence-Based Physical Activity Programs for Older Adults into Community Settings." *American Journal of Public Health,* 2006, *96,* 1201–1209.
9. Strictly speaking, the Robert Wood Johnson Foundation makes the award, based on the recommendations of National Program Office and National Advisory Committee.

CHAPTER 7

The Urban Health Initiative

Paul S. Jellinek

Editors' Introduction

From the draft riots of the 1860s to the racial riots of the 1960s, urban violence has signaled major problems in American society. In 1992, Rodney King, an African-American, was beaten by Los Angeles police officers after a traffic stop. The beating was recorded on video. The acquittal of the accused police officers triggered a riot in which fifty-five people were killed, more than two thousand were injured, and the damage to property was extensive. This riot led to congressional hearings, and it forced government agencies and foundations trying to improve social and economic conditions to reexamine their work in America's cities.

Prior to the Los Angeles riots, the Robert Wood Johnson Foundation had awarded few large grants to improve health in inner cities. A result of the post-1992 reexamination was the development of the Urban Health Initiative, a major effort to improve the health and safety of children living in five medium-size and large cities. What made the Urban Health Initiative unusual was its commitment to improving the health of a significant number of children in the five cities. It was not just a pilot project or a demonstration to test new approaches;

rather, the Urban Health Initiative was a program with the ambitious goal of making a positive difference in the cities' health statistics—in effect, undertaking a role usually played by government.

The chapter raises an interesting and important question: how can foundations fund programs of sufficient size to improve the health of a significant number of people living in distressed urban areas? The resources of foundations, after all, pale in comparison to those of government. The Robert Wood Johnson Foundation, the nation's fourth-largest foundation, awards between $400 million and $500 million a year in a $2 trillion health economy. The annual budget of the City of Los Angeles is $6.7 billion.

This question of scale led the Urban Health Initiative to create what it called *the denominator exercise,* which asks (1) How many kids are in need of help? (the denominator) and (2) What will it take to have an impact of a substantial percentage of those kids? This exercise provides an indication of the size of the effort required to have an impact.

Paul Jellinek, the author of this chapter, played an important role in the development of the Urban Health Initiative when he was a vice president at the Robert Wood Johnson Foundation. This chapter provides Jellinek, now a partner in a consulting firm that advises foundations, an opportunity to take a retrospective look at a program that he helped launch over a decade ago.

"My aunt and uncle in Detroit who raised me didn't speak any English, so I never had any help with school when I came here from Puerto Rico," recalls Luis Cartagena, a single father who still lives in Detroit. Luis, who has silver hair and a gentle smile, is now raising his six-year-old son, Adam. "I don't read or write, and I have been on my own since I was sixteen," he says. "I have been surviving my way through life. Because of that, I knew I would have a hard time educating Adam. I needed help—and I got it, from Latino Family Services and its summer and after-school programs.

"Adam has been through a lot," Luis continues. "I thought if I could get him around a group of children his age, that would be good for him. He looks forward to coming to the after-school program. He is here"—at Latino Family Services—"from 3:30 until 6:00 five days a week. He has a chance to learn things, to be social, and to pick up skills. He plays on a computer. The staff helps him with his reading and homework; they do arts and crafts and take the children on field trips. The program has helped interest him in learning, and he has learned how to get along with other children. His behavior has dramatically changed since coming here."

Luis pauses. "If this place wasn't here, I wouldn't have known what to do," he says. "I'd be lost. This place gives him a better chance to succeed than I had."[1]

This is the kind of good news that one hears all too rarely in media stories about big cities like Detroit. Yet what may be most significant about Adam's story is not simply that he wound up in an after-school program that his father believes has changed his life. It is that, according to recent statistics collected by Mayor's Time—a nonprofit organization based in Detroit and funded by the Robert Wood Johnson Foundation through its Urban Health Initiative—the chance of a school-aged child in Detroit finding and getting into such a program in the first place is today more than double what it was six years ago, when Adam was born.

In 1999, it was estimated that only one in five school-aged children in Detroit was involved in after-school activities. By 2006, Mayor's Time reports, that number had jumped to more than 50 percent. And Detroit's annual After-School Fair, which began in 2001 and enrolled thirty thousand children in after-school programs over its first four years, signed up thirty-one thousand more children in 2006 alone. An increase of that magnitude, with its potential to improve the health and safety—and ultimately the life chances—of tens of thousands of Detroit's children is indeed good news, not only for Detroit but also for other cities across the country struggling to make a better life for their children.

Sometimes the Cards Are Stacked Against Big Cities

The dramatic increase in after-school enrollment in Detroit was brought about through the hard work of many individuals and organizations, but a pivotal part of the story can be traced back to an event that occurred more than a decade earlier and more than two thousand miles away: the Los Angeles riots of 1992. Sparked by the Rodney King verdict, the riots sent shock waves across the nation, all the way to Washington, D.C., where Congress convened hearings to try to understand what had happened and to determine what might be done to prevent such outbreaks in the future, both in Los Angeles and elsewhere.

On the roster of expert witnesses were several foundation presidents, including Steven Schroeder, president of the Robert Wood Johnson Foundation. In preparing his testimony, Schroeder, who had joined the Foundation just two years earlier, was startled to discover that although the Foundation had made many grants to urban organizations and institutions since becoming a national philanthropy in 1972, the nation's largest cities—including Los Angeles—were notably underrepresented. Moreover, it appeared that few of the Foundation's grants that *had* been awarded in the largest cities were of sufficient scale or duration to have had more than a marginal impact on the immense problems and health challenges facing those cities.

This finding was echoed in a report prepared for the Foundation by Charles Royer, the former mayor of Seattle, which noted that the Foundation tended "to gravitate toward the same cities" in many of its competitive national programs, and that "sometimes the cards are stacked against big cities because of the difficulty of making a difference with the amount of money available."

Following his appearance before Congress, Schroeder called a meeting of the Foundation's program staff. He expressed his concern that the Foundation hadn't been doing enough to help the nation's largest and most distressed cities, and he challenged the staff to come up with fresh ideas for a program that would help those cities tackle some of their most urgent health needs.

The Federal Spigot Was Being Turned Off

It was a tough challenge. For one thing, since the mid-1980s, the Foundation's major programs in areas of concern to cities, such as homelessness, mental illness, AIDS, and substance abuse, had called for collaboration among the key players in the funded communities, primarily because most of these problems were too big and too complex for any single agency or institution to deal with on its own. But getting local grassroots AIDS agencies to collaborate with the one public hospital in Dallas or New Orleans was one thing; fostering the same kind of collaboration with New York City's *nineteen* public hospitals was an entirely different ballgame.

Of course, one approach to working with larger cities might be to focus on a section of the city rather than trying to take on the city as a whole. This was what the Foundation had been doing with some of the larger cities in Fighting Back, its program to reduce demand for illegal drugs and alcohol.[2] However, as the staff was learning from its experience with the Fighting Back program, a subsection of a larger city by itself often didn't have the political clout to bring about the kinds of policy changes needed to make any headway.

Meanwhile, at the national level, a development with potentially profound implications was taking shape: the federal government, faced with record budget deficits, was beginning to cut back sharply on spending for new health and social programs. This went to the heart of what, until then, had been the Robert Wood Johnson Foundation's principal strategy for bringing about large-scale change—big national demonstration programs designed to test new ways of delivering health services, especially to the poor and underserved. The idea was that if these new ways of delivering health care proved to be effective, the federal government would step in with the resources necessary to replicate the approach nationwide. Recent examples included the replication of the Foundation's program of health care for the homeless through the McKinney Act, and the replication of its AIDS health services program through the Ryan White Act.

But now the federal spigot was being turned off. Not only did this knock the legs out from under the Foundation's demonstration and replication strategy for leveraging social change, but it also left the nation's cities to fend for themselves as they tried to get their arms around a dizzying array of health and social problems.

The Health and Safety of Children

In 1992, I was a program vice president at the Robert Wood Johnson Foundation. On June 22, 1992, less than three months after the Los Angeles riots and shortly after Steven Schroeder's challenge to the Foundation's staff to come up with a new program specifically for the nation's big cities, I sent a memo to Richard Reynolds, who was then the Foundation's executive vice president, suggesting that the Foundation begin to develop a major, long-term Foundation initiative to secure the health and safety of children in some of the nation's biggest cities.

The memo recommended that the initiative should "deliberately target our biggest cities" and that its length should be nine or ten years—more than double the four-year life of the Foundation's typical national demonstration program. It also recommended getting policymakers involved at the outset, and urged that close attention be given to the role of the media, because public awareness and support would be essential to the ultimate success of the initiative.

Reynolds liked the idea and suggested that those on the staff interested in pursuing it should form an informal working group to do the necessary groundwork and prepare a paper for discussion by the full staff. The result was a thirteen-member staff working group on urban health. It was chaired initially by Ruby Hearn, then a Foundation vice president, and later by Rush Russell, at the time a senior program officer at the Foundation.

A Different Program Design

The members of the working group began by immersing themselves in the literature—wading through stacks of books, journals, evaluation reports, conference proceedings, and foundation papers. They then fanned out across the country, meeting with a diverse array of academics, policy experts, experienced practitioners, and staff members from other foundations that had a track record in the urban arena, including Annie E. Casey, Ford, Rockefeller, Pew, and Sierra Health.

As a result of this background work, Hearn and Russell became convinced that if this new urban initiative was to be successful, it would need a different program design. "We were not aiming to replicate a promising model as in many previous Foundation programs," Hearn recalls. "We had learned that substantial changes of the kind we envisioned would require a level of political will that could result only from broad community engagement."

Over the next several months, as the new initiative began to take shape, some of its key distinguishing features emerged:

- A more rigorous site selection process than usual, including in-depth reconnaissance and analysis up front to assess the readiness of each candidate city to undertake the initiative.
- A commitment by the Foundation of up to ten years.
- A citywide focus, even in the biggest cities, that would reach tens of thousands of children or more. This, it was believed, would elicit greater local political support for the initiative than if the focus were limited to a relatively small section of the city.
- A regional strategy through which the cities would try to enlist the involvement of suburbs and other communities in their region to obtain the necessary support and cooperation at the county, state, and federal levels.

- Local self-determination—meaning that the cities would decide for themselves what specific children's health issue they wanted to tackle. This contrasted with the traditional demonstration program, in which the participating sites were generally replicating a prescribed model to address a common problem.
- Communications as an active intervention in its own right, rather than simply a public relations tool—both to generate public support for the necessary systems changes and as a means of promoting positive health behavior.

Ultimately, it was the emphasis on the large-scale expansion of services that lay at the heart of this new initiative and that most sharply distinguished it from most of the Foundation's past programs. No longer was it sufficient for a Foundation program simply to serve a couple of hundred young people in a model clinic in the hope that the model would be picked up and "taken to scale" by the federal government. Now the program itself would have to do the heavy lifting, helping cities to figure out new ways to reach very large numbers of at-risk children and youth—in fact, enough children to change the health statistics for the city as a whole—*without* a major infusion of new federal dollars. In most cases, that would mean using existing dollars that were already in the system in sometimes radically new and more effective ways. And that, it soon became clear, represented a whole new programmatic paradigm, both for the Foundation and for the grantees.

Fraught with Risk

In the fall of 1994, the working group presented a detailed twenty-eight-page report describing the proposed new initiative to the full program staff. After a lively debate about whether the idea was *too* big, a proposal for a new urban health initiative was drafted and presented to the board of trustees. In January of 1995, the board authorized an initial three-year, $4 million grant to get the program off the ground in up to five cities.

With the authorization in place, the staff working group quickly assembled a team of senior consultants from around the country with expertise in urban health and policy to assist it in identifying the most promising cities in which to carry out the initiative. A list of twenty potential sites was drawn up; it included major cities such as New York, Chicago, and Philadelphia, as well as some smaller distressed cities such as Oakland, California, and Richmond, Virginia.

Next, detailed statistical profiles of each of the twenty cities were prepared, press coverage from each city was carefully reviewed to get a sense of current local priorities and the local political climate, and calls were made to knowledgeable observers in each city who could provide an honest assessment of the local leadership's capacity and its potential interest in an initiative of this kind. Based on these preliminary assessments, teams of staff and consultants visited many of the cities on the list, meeting with key officials and community leaders to get a better sense of their record of local collaboration and their appetite for a major new initiative to improve the health and safety of their city's children.

In May, a letter went out over Steven Schroeder's signature to leaders in these cities inviting them to apply for two years of development funding under the program, which at that point was called America's Promise. (In 1997, the name was changed to the Urban Health Initiative, after a Presidents' Summit chaired by Colin Powell adopted the name "America's Promise" for its national youth initiative.) After an intensive review process, eight cities—Baltimore, Chicago, Detroit, Miami, Oakland, Philadelphia, Richmond, and Sacramento—were awarded two-year development grants, with the understanding that after the first two years, up to five of them would receive substantial additional support to help implement the initiative for a period of up to eight years.*

*Ironically, given Los Angeles' role in sparking the initiative, that city was not included. It was still very much preoccupied with extensive rebuilding in the aftermath of the riots, and the Foundation had already provided separate funding to Los Angeles to support health services planning as part of the rebuilding effort.

Lost in All of the Process Details

Charles Royer, the former Seattle mayor, whose report had helped to make the case for a special focus on big cities, had been among the group of senior consultants who had helped the Foundation select the eight cities, and he now agreed to serve as the initiative's national program director. This meant that he and his staff, operating out of a national program office to be established at the University of Washington in Seattle, would manage the initiative on a day-to-day basis and would provide technical assistance and direction to the grantees.

Right off the bat, there were problems. Because of various processing delays, by the time the university actually received the funding from the Foundation to set up the office and hire a staff, the eight cities had already had their grants for a month, and a number of them were in dire need of technical assistance. As the National Program Office's first annual report to the Foundation drily noted, "The sites were funded January 1, 1996. The National Program Office was funded a month later. As a result, the time normally used to refine programmatic ideas and approaches, develop systems to assist sites and monitor grants, plan major activities, and establish administrative functions was eliminated."

The delay in setting up the National Program Office was not the only problem. The fact that the eight cities would be competing for five much bigger implementation grants just two years down the road made some of them reluctant to ask for help, afraid that such a request would be taken as a sign of weakness. By the same token, Royer and his staff sometimes found themselves holding back on providing the level of technical assistance that they felt was needed, because they didn't want to appear to be favoring one city over another while the cities were locked in competition with one another.

But the biggest problem, it soon became apparent, was that a lot of people simply did not understand the initiative. Specifically, what wasn't sufficiently clear at that point was the *scale* of the Foundation's vision: to reach enough young people with effective interventions to change the child health statistics for the city as a whole. That meant serving thousands, or even tens of thousands, of children in each city. Looking back, Royer observes, "That was the biggest piece of the initiative, and the most attractive. But it got lost in all of the process details early on. So people didn't really realize it until later."

The Denominator Exercise

One immediate result of this misunderstanding was that most of the cities initially hired the wrong people to serve as project directors. Although many of the project directors had extensive hands-on experience working in their communities, few had worked on the kind of large-scale systems change that this initiative was all about. Consequently, most of them didn't understand the kinds of influential people they would need on their boards or the kinds of data that would have to be collected. Nor did they understand why it was so critical that they develop "the right connections," both within their region and with officials in state government, or why the Foundation kept insisting on the importance of developing a sophisticated communications strategy. The upshot of all of this was that the Foundation and the eight cities spent much of the first two years talking past each other, with the National Program Office caught somewhere in between.

The turning point, recalls Cynthia Curreri, the program's deputy director, came during a site visit to Chicago near the end of the second year. "The police chief came in, and went on about this program he was going to do that sounded wonderful, and then [someone on the site visit team] says, 'How many kids will you be able to get to, Chief?' And the chief says, 'Eighty-five,' or whatever the number was. And suddenly I realized, 'OK, this isn't going to work. That's never going to make a meaningful difference in a city the size of Chicago.' So that was the moment when it really all came together for me—that one question to the chief. And that's when I decided that we had to have a way for people to work out how many kids they would have to get to in order to make it worthwhile. We had to have some way for them to put numbers to it."

As soon as Curreri returned to the office in Seattle, she began drafting what came to be known as the denominator exercise, a quantitative tool to help the project directors calculate just how many of their city's children they would need to reach in order to have a real impact on the citywide statistic for the particular health problem they were trying to address. What's more, by plugging in the cost per child of the chosen intervention, they could calculate how much money it would take to get there.

Ramping Up

As the first two years came to an end, the eight cities submitted their proposals for implementation funding. Following another round of intensive review, five of them—Baltimore, Detroit, Oakland, Philadelphia, and Richmond—were selected.[†] Given the small number, they were a surprisingly diverse group, not only in size and geography but also in terms of where their projects were housed. Richmond's project, for example, was run by the Greater Richmond Chamber of Commerce, whereas Philadelphia's was based—at least initially—in city government.

Although these five cities now had sizeable implementation grants to carry them for the next four years, with the possibility of an additional four-year renewal, they were hardly home free. The implementation grants came with significant conditions attached, including, in several cases, the need for new leadership with a better grasp of the dynamics of large-scale systems change. Moreover, all of the cities still had a good deal of work to do on their denominator exercises before they would finally be in a position to put hard numbers to their goals and begin developing realistic strategies for achieving them.

In the meantime, both the Foundation and the National Program Office began ramping up their own efforts to support and learn from the initiative. The Foundation had funded Beth Weitzman and Diana Silver, two experienced researchers at New York University's Robert F. Wagner Graduate School of Public Service, to plan an independent evaluation of the initiative. In addition, Ruby Hearn and James Knickman, then the

---

[†]In April 1997, the Foundation awarded $24 million over two years to implement the Urban Health Initiative. Four years later, it awarded another $24 million. Additionally, the Foundation authorized funds to enable the National Program Office to manage the program.

Foundation's vice president for research and evaluation, wanted to create an ongoing forum that would bring the Urban Health Initiative grantees together with leading scholars in the field. "We believed that it was crucial to promote a dialogue between academics studying community change and practitioners trying to bring about such changes so that they could learn from one another as the initiative unfolded," Hearn recalls. "We were very fortunate to enlist the help of William Julius Wilson, the country's leading urban researcher, to develop and conduct the seminar series at Harvard University."

The National Program Office, which felt liberated to provide much more extensive guidance and technical assistance now that the cities were no longer in competition, also came up with a number of ways to inspire and support the often beleaguered project directors and their staffs. For example, Royer and his staff set up an urban fellowship program in each city to engage a cross-section of local leaders—such as judges, business leaders, and journalists—in the initiative. And every year Royer would take a group of leaders from each of the five cities on a so-called "Inter-City Leadership Visit" to a city outside the Urban Health Initiative that was doing something especially innovative or relevant to the initiative. Finally, to assist and advise the Foundation and the National Program Office as well as the cities themselves, a National Advisory Committee of experts in health, urban policy, and youth development was assembled, several of whom became deeply committed to helping the cities succeed.

The first step for each site was to determine on which specific aspects of children's health and safety to focus. Although existing health statistics were clearly an important part of the process, it was also essential to hear what local leaders and local residents—including the city's young people themselves—had to say. Otherwise, as past experience had shown, there wouldn't be sufficient buy-in for the initiative to succeed. All five of the sites reached out to their communities to elicit their views, but the Baltimore project went perhaps the furthest, convening some seven thousand city residents in a spirited public meeting that generated more than thirty initial priorities for improving the health and safety of the city's children—an extraordinarily ambitious list that eventually had to be whittled down to a more manageable number. As a result of the data and the public input they had received, most of the sites identified the reduction of youth violence as one of their top priorities, with reductions in substance abuse and teen pregnancy not far behind. Several sites also wanted to improve birth outcomes and school readiness and to reduce child abuse and neglect.

The next step for the sites was to determine what kinds of interventions were out there that they could use to tackle these problems. In particular, they were looking for programs and policies that had been evaluated and had been shown to be effective—preferably with hard numbers documenting just *how* effective and at what cost.

After-school programs turned out to be a popular choice at almost every site. Nurse home visiting services for pregnant teenagers and their children—which had been found to improve birth outcomes, reduce child abuse, and delay subsequent pregnancies—were another popular option, as was an intensive interagency homicide reduction program that had first been developed in Boston several years earlier. Richmond, taking the long view, decided to focus on having all of its children reading at grade level by the time they entered the third grade—which, the research suggested, was a powerful way to reduce pregnancy rates during the teenage years.

With their interventions in hand, together with the basic statistics on the number of children in their city who had the particular problem that they had decided to target, the sites were ready to start working on Curreri's denominator exercise. Largely because of difficulties in understanding the exercise or its utility, as well as challenges in obtaining the necessary local data, this proved much harder than expected. But with the pain came some important gains. "Sites that moved on [the denominator exercise] quickly and completed the exercise for the first strategies being implemented—Richmond, Baltimore, Philadelphia—were very surprised at the results," the National Program Office's third annual report recounts. "All three [sites] have significantly modified their plans based on the information gained. Richmond phased implementation of [its] strategies and dropped one altogether . . . Baltimore phased implementation and set up a whole new committee system to trace and plan how to realign and increase resources upon learning the frightening cost of their initial strategies. Philadelphia expanded outside its initial 'target areas' for two strategies and is considering dropping a third on learning what they must do to achieve scale."

In other words, once the city projects had worked their way through the denominator exercise, the result was some pretty serious sticker shock among the project directors and their boards. "That's when the light went on for a lot of them: when they saw that it was maybe going to take hundreds of millions of dollars—way more money than they had in their grants," Curreri recalls. "And so what's their strategy? What services can be identified that are currently being funded but that aren't doing a good job, and how can they get that money moved from one place to another—which requires a very heavy political strategy? That's really the main story of the Urban Health Initiative."

Although the sites hoped to raise at least some new money from the government and from the private sector, they quickly realized that to fund effective programs at the level needed to achieve "scale," they would have to persuade the major public and private funders to redirect some of the vast sums of money that were already in the system for children toward these programs—and that would indeed require a substantial political strategy.

And so their next step was to determine how much money was actually being spent in each city for children—all of it, both public and private—and to ascertain precisely where the money came from, who controlled it, and what the particular constraints were on each of the myriad funding streams that went to children's services. As Royer told the project directors, "You have to find the one person in your city who really understands the guts of the budget, and get to be their best friend." Ernest Jones, the longtime chair of Philadelphia Safe and Sound, which runs the Urban Health Initiative in that city, points out that "prior to Safe and Sound, nobody knew how much the city spent for children's services."[3]

Then came the truly challenging part: using the numbers to try to educate both policymakers and the public to make the system "work smarter for kids," as Royer put it. Philadelphia Safe and Sound, for example, made the results of its budget analysis public, holding a press conference and issuing a "report card" each year that presented the most recent data on juvenile crime, teen pregnancy, and other key indicators, together with a "children's budget" that showed how all the money in the system for children was actually being spent. By making these kinds of data public and pointing out some of the obvious misalignments between where the needs were and where the resources were going, the sites eventually helped to bring about the reallocation of hundreds of millions of existing dollars toward more effective interventions.

Money wasn't the only issue. The sites also paid close attention to nonfinancial resources—such as the hundreds of school buildings that often stood empty during the after-school hours. Recognizing that there was no conceivable way that the cities could afford to build all of the new facilities that would be required to provide after-school programs to large numbers of additional children, the sites, using their data and working with key partners in their cities, were eventually able to bring about changes in school policies and to break through long-standing barriers that had kept the schools closed to after-school activities. The Baltimore, Detroit, Oakland, and Philadelphia sites, for example, negotiated agreements with their local school districts that allowed private and community organizations to make their programs available to children within school buildings during nonschool hours. As the National Program Office noted, "These arrangements . . . were critical to achieving scale, as expansion could not occur without access to low cost, or no cost, physical plants in which to operate."

Despite the assistance and the hundreds of thousands of dollars they received each year from the Foundation, these five projects were, in fact, very small Davids going up against some enormous Goliaths. As Diana Silver, of the evaluation team, notes, "They were up against people who were deeply invested in not having those policies, [including] certain principals and others in the school system, as well as . . . people who would no longer be able to dole out favors the way they had in the past." This conflict took a toll. "I can't tell you how many times I had people in tears on the phone," Cynthia Curreri recalls. "They were just so frustrated, and they'd say, 'I just can't do this another day. It's so *hard*.'"

Five Sites, Five Approaches, and Many Common Challenges

As the five Urban Health Initiative grantees strengthened their analytic capacity and expanded their networks of relationships, they gradually established themselves as trusted intermediaries, committed to improving the health and safety of their cities' children by deploying existing resources more effectively. Among their activities:

- Baltimore's Safe & Sound Campaign spearheaded the creation of a citywide data collaborative to keep track of what was happening to the city's children and leveraged more than $10 million a year in public and private funds to support its strategies. With the data and additional resources, Safe & Sound worked with agencies in the city to develop a comprehensive array of initiatives, including the Success by 6 Partnership, which helps families with young children to prepare them to succeed in school; Reading by Nine, a program in the school system to increase the number of students reading at grade level by age nine; Operation Safe Kids, a partnership between law enforcement and public health officials to provide high-risk young people with intensive case management (as an alternative to incarceration); and a variety of after-school programs.
- In Detroit, Mayor's Time raised millions of dollars from government, foundations, and the business community in support of its after-school strategy; worked closely with the Skillman Foundation and state and city agencies to secure federal funding for free breakfasts and lunches for young people participating in summer programs; and secured an agreement from city government to invest $400 million of casino tax revenues to improve and expand recreation center physical plants and activities over the next ten years. In addition, Mayor's Time developed a citywide information system, which for the first time began collecting youth participation and outcome data from hundreds of after-school providers,

and launched an interactive Web site to enable parents and children throughout the city to identify after-school opportunities available in their neighborhoods.

- Oakland's Safe Passages brought together senior officials from city and county government, the school district, and community-based organizations in an unprecedented collaborative effort to provide the full range of supportive services needed by the city's at-risk children and adolescents. Major components included an early intervention program to promote reading, language skills, and positive social interaction among preschool children; a case management and mental health program for at-risk middle school students; an after-school strategy; and Pathways to Change, a program that provided intensive case management to repeat youth offenders. Violence-related school suspensions declined by 78 percent in one year among students in the Pathways to Change program.[4]

- In addition to its annual Report Card and Children's Budget, Philadelphia Safe and Sound created an online after-school and child-care program finder, which provides information on more than seven hundred programs, and began developing an ambitious integrated data system to improve the coordination and delivery of services for the tens of thousands of at-risk children and adolescents served by city agencies. Also, as a result of Safe and Sound's efforts, nearly $80 million a year in new and redirected funds was raised in support of an array of services that included nurse home visiting for pregnant teenage mothers, life skills training for at-risk youth, youth violence reduction, and expanded after-school programs.

- In Richmond, Youth Matters began with the specific goal of ensuring that by 2010 all of the city's children would be reading at or above grade level by the time they reached the third grade. Subsequently, Youth Matters helped to create a 150-member coalition to increase the availability and im-

> prove the quality of early childhood development programs throughout Richmond. As a result of these efforts, home visiting services have been provided to at-risk children, and many of the city's young children are receiving improved preschool services. In addition, a book bank created by the coalition to help improve reading readiness has distributed eighty-five thousand books since 2001.[5]

Most of these accomplishments did not come easily. In Richmond, James Dunn, president of the Chamber of Commerce, which housed Youth Matters, recalls, "Getting the different stakeholders—elected officials, school boards—to the table and getting them to put the interests of the kids first—that took a lot longer than I would have thought. There was lots of caution, lots of skepticism, and lots of suspicion. Everybody was asking each other, 'What are *you* trying to get out of this?'"

Compounding the problem of mutual mistrust was the fact that key players in the system kept changing. Naomi Post, who ran Safe and Sound in Philadelphia for several years, points out that over the course of the initiative, the Philadelphia School District went through a state takeover and had three different superintendents. This constant turnover, she says, required "continuous engagement with different leaders, with varying priorities, to ensure the sustainability of services based in public schools." In fact, the same kind of continual turnover was occurring in all five cities—not just with school superintendents but also with mayors, city managers, police chiefs, health and human service commissioners, city council members, county commissioners, and others.

Then, of course, there was the economy, which had been in reasonably good shape during the first few years of the initiative but started going downhill in 2001. Judge Freddie Burton, Jr., who chairs the board of Mayor's Time in Detroit, puts it bluntly: "Our biggest challenge has been money. We here in Michigan are experiencing some major downturns in our major industry, and that has slowed us down. We have achieved our goal of 50 percent participation [in after-school activities], but I wish we could get closer to 100 percent. There is still such a need."

Summing Up

After a decade of activities, what has the Urban Health Initiative accomplished?

In its final report to the Foundation in early 2006, the National Program Office offered this statistical summary:

> Though sites varied in their success, four of the five final sites either achieved scale in one or more of their strategies or demonstrated that they were on a trajectory to reach scale within a reasonable period of time. Detroit's Mayor's Time, at the end of ten years, will have reached over 40,000 young people in its after-school strategy. Baltimore's Safe & Sound Campaign reached nearly 3,000 families with home visitation and center-based care, and its after-school strategy reached nearly 24,000 young people. Philadelphia Safe and Sound reached over 45,000 young people with its after-school effort, and about 600 with its Youth Violence Reduction Partnership, which targeted a small number of particularly high-risk offenders. Oakland's Safe Passages achieved or exceeded scale in two of its strategies, after-school activities for middle school youth and integration of mental health services into the school day. Richmond's Youth Matters, the only site failing to demonstrate adequate movement toward scale, still reached nearly 10,000 children with enhanced teaching experiences as a result of its strategy to improve the quality of preschool.

In other words, according to the National Program Office, four of the five sites had either reached, or were within striking distance of reaching, enough children in their cities with effective interventions to make a substantial dent in their "denominators."

Whether this will translate into a corresponding improvement in the cities' child health statistics remains an open question—in part because, as the National Program Office notes, it could take several years of sustained service at scale to significantly change outcomes, and in part because the kinds of health outcomes that the sites were targeting—youth violence, substance abuse, teen pregnancy, child abuse and neglect—are ultimately subject to a wide range of influences that lie beyond the control of the sites. Not the least of these, according to the evaluation team, is the extensive migration both into and out of the five cities over the ten years of the Urban Health Initiative, meaning that any changes in city health statistics that are detected may have more to do with changes in the population than with the impact of any specific interventions.

In addition to programmatic activities, the sites have leveraged a considerable amount of money. "In total," according to the National Program Office, "the sites report that they will have succeeded in establishing continuing investments in their strategies of well over $200 million annually." If this level of funding is maintained over time, it will represent an impressive rate of return on the $65 million that the Robert Wood Johnson Foundation invested in the Urban Health Initiative over a ten-year period.

Perhaps as important as the amount is the fact that much of this leveraged money is being redirected into prevention services—a change that, as the National Program Office notes, "was not an easy task." In Philadelphia, for example, the share of the city's human services budget dedicated to prevention rose from 2 percent to 13 percent between 1999 and 2006; actual expenditures rose from $7.8 million to $85.2 million, more than a tenfold increase. Moreover, Philadelphia Safe and Sound played a major role in securing an agreement that requires two of the city's professional sports teams—the Phillies and the Eagles—each to donate a million dollars a year to a children's fund for the next thirty years.

Baltimore, meanwhile, has negotiated an agreement with its state government, called the Maryland Opportunity Compact, which, according to Safe & Sound executive director Hathaway Ferebee, "is a new financing and accountability tool that redirects funding away from custodial programs to interventions that produce positive results," such as the provision of intensive case management services for foster care children whose parents have substance abuse problems. Based on a model program in San Diego, this case management approach is expected to reduce the average length of stay in foster care, yielding savings to the state of as much as $30,000 per child.

The numbers and the dollars, however, are not the whole story. In the cities themselves, those close to the Urban Health Initiative see its effects as highly positive. In Oakland, David Kears—who, as the county's long-time health director, has been involved from the beginning—sees its greatest accomplishment as "the true integration of the city, the county, and the schools—especially the schools—not only within [the Urban Health Initiative] but also beyond." In Detroit, Judge Freddie Burton says that the initiative "is galvanizing a partnership across lines, whether it be racial lines, ethnic lines—whatever." Grenaé Dudley, the project's executive director in Detroit since 1998, adds that after many years of widespread reluctance to become involved in after-school programming, "this year every Detroit public school was at the After-School Fair—all 280 schools!" Douglas Nelson, president of the Annie E. Casey Foundation, notes that "prior to the work of the Safe & Sound Campaign [in Baltimore] there was neither a centralized nor an accessible data source to inform public policy and public and private investments on behalf of children, youth, and families."

The evaluation team, which has not yet completed its work, offers its own preliminary assessment of the initiative. In brief summary, the evaluators found that the Urban Health Initiative had had a measurable but modest impact in its major areas of focus. "None of these cities have been totally turned around by the Urban Health Initiative," says Beth Weitzman, the principal investigator on the evaluation (which had not been published as this book went to press). However, she continues, "There is concrete evidence that each of the sites did achieve some tangible changes in the way business was being done, and some of them are remarkable, especially given the way that the economy tanked in 2001. Oakland, for instance, has really gotten into this sort of blending of funds, and thinking creatively about funding. We interviewed the new head of juvenile justice there . . . and he said the strangest thing for him was that he would go to a meeting with a problem like truancy, and the school system person and the health department person would each say, 'OK, well, I think I can kick in this much toward that.' He said he'd never seen anything like it before—and he was someone who'd been around."

Finally, there is the perspective of Harvard's William Julius Wilson, whose seminar series brought together the ground troops of the Urban Health Initiative with some of the nation's leading urban researchers in an ongoing dialogue: "The Urban Health Initiative provides us with a unique opportunity to better understand how a focus on the organizational infrastructure of social service systems can produce lasting improvements in the way that cities address residents' health and safety issues. Through the work of effective intermediaries who function as critical buffers between policymakers and the people they serve, the Urban Health Initiative model warrants serious consideration as a mechanism for tackling complex problems."

In the end, what do all of these numbers and all of these changes in complex urban financing and service delivery systems add up to at a human level? Simply stated, they mean that genuine positive change *is* possible, even in some of our most distressed cities, and that Luis Cartagena's son, Adam—along with many thousands of children like him in the five cities of the Urban Health Initiative—does have a better chance than his father had to be healthy and safe and to succeed in life.

Notes

1. Larson, T., Sanoff, A., and Ellis, M. "Five Cities Are Improving the Odds For Their Children: Here's How." Seattle, Wash.: Urban Health Institute National Program Office, Institute for Community Change, 11.
2. Wielawski, I. "The Fighting Back Program." *To Improve Health and Health Care, Vol. VII: The Robert Wood Johnson Foundation Anthology.* San Francisco: Jossey-Bass, 2004.
3. Larson, Sanoff, and Ellis, 11.
4. Larson, Sanoff, and Ellis, 12.
5. Larson, Sanoff, and Ellis, 20.

CHAPTER 8

Mentoring Young People

Irene M. Wielawski

Editors' Introduction

The importance of a caring adult in the life of a child cannot be overstated, yet one out of five young people—or 8.5 million kids—lacks a caring adult presence in his or her life.[1] Ideally, that adult is a parent or close relative, but in many cases that caring adult is not a family member, but a mentor. That mentor may be a teacher at school, a staff member at a Boys and Girls Club, a coach from a Police Activities League team, a volunteer from a program such as Big Brothers Big Sisters, or a neighborhood friend. Where a mentor comes from is not critical. What *is* critical is that a child has an adult in his or her life who can provide guidance, values, stability, and love.

Although mentoring has never been a high priority of the Robert Wood Johnson Foundation, the Foundation has, nonetheless, invested more than $29 million to support it since 1989. These investments have taken a variety of forms. They include research to better understand the concept of positive youth development and to explore the factors that lead children living in disadvantaged, often dangerous, circumstances to tap their underlying resiliency and to thrive. Mainly, however, they include programs that test different approaches to bringing caring adults into the lives of at-risk children—from volunteer and paid mentors to after-school sports programs.

In this chapter, Irene Wielawski examines both the research on mentoring and the Foundation-funded programs to encourage it. Wielawski, a frequent contributor to the *Anthology* series, is an award-winning health care journalist. She has been a medical writer for the *Providence Journal-Bulletin* and the *Los Angeles Times.*

Notes

1. America's Promise Alliance. Every Child, Every Promise. (http://www.americaspromise.org/uploadedFiles/AmericasPromiseAlliance/Every_Child_Every_Promise/ECEP_Reports_-_JPEG/ECEP%20-%20Full%20Report.pdf)

—₩— Look at the cover of the *New York Times* Sunday magazine from September 24, 2006. You'll see a photo of nine men and women—young and old—posing on a football field. Everyone is looking straight at the camera, but the viewer's eye is drawn to the young man in a red football jersey in the background. He is Michael Oher, star left tackle for the University of Mississippi and the subject of the article, standing straddle-legged and impassive, helmet in hand, in the classic pose of a gridiron superstar.

But what are all these other people doing in the photo? There's a cheerleader, a young boy in a red Ole Miss T-shirt, a mom type, and some men. The hint of what the article will reveal lies in a crosshatch of hand-drawn arrows leading from Oher to everyone else, then meandering among them before arching back to Oher.

If the emerging health field concerned with the functional well-being of children were reduced to a pictograph, this would be the tell-all image—a diagram of the critically important relationships with adults and peers that help children grow into confident, ethical, and socially competent people.

The accompanying article details how everyone in the cover photo contributed to the rescue of Oher, the neglected and often homeless child of a murdered father and a crack-addicted mother.[1] The circumstances of his early life are not unique. What makes Oher's story newsworthy is his astonishing trajectory from street urchin who barely knew what it was to sleep in a bed to multimillion-dollar pro football prospect.

Sadly, most children born into extreme poverty and whipsawed by family turmoil don't get rescued. The statistics on these children—called "disadvantaged" by social scientists—are grim. Many don't finish high school, and significant numbers of them end up in the juvenile justice system. Statistically, they're at greater risk for substance abuse and early pregnancy. Experts say they are more likely to die young, victims of violence, drug overdose, or accident.

It's a bleak picture, but not hopeless. Within this population of children are some who find their way out of the mayhem and go on to lead stable and productive lives. How do they do it? Interested in this question, a handful of social scientists began to study these children in the early 1990s—to identify factors that helped them succeed, rather than to pursue the traditional inquiry into why children fail. Slowly they began to identify characteristics—called protective factors—that give children added resiliency in the face of adversity. Intelligence is one of these factors; children of higher than average intellectual ability, researchers say, are better able to navigate harmful environments while also reaping valuable psychic benefits from school success. Another protective factor is having positive and caring relationships with adults.

The research underpinning these theories is still relatively new. But it is the foundation of an emerging field called *positive youth development,* which seeks to buttress children's natural resiliency and, especially during the adolescent years, help them steer clear of alcohol and drug abuse, truancy, criminal behavior, and early pregnancy.[2] Between 1997 and 2000, the Robert Wood Johnson Foundation supported the research of the Columbia University professor Jeanne Brooks-Gunn and her colleagues into youth-development programs and their effectiveness in reducing risky behavior.[3] This emphasis on the prevention of unhealthy choices captured the interest of the Robert Wood Johnson Foundation, which in recent years has funded a number of experiments to improve options for disadvantaged children.

Two of these experiments—Friends of the Children and the After School Project—illustrate opposite ends of a broad range of initiatives to improve the social health of children. Friends of the Children is an intensive, long-term mentoring program that works one-on-one with youngsters from kindergarten through high school. Founded in Portland, Oregon, in 1993, it is the brainchild of a local entrepreneur and philanthropist whose commitment—and practical understanding of the needs of disadvantaged children—stems from his own bleak childhood. The After School Project sought to embed positive youth development principles into existing public, private, paid, and volunteer after-school programs in three cities. Acting in a less direct manner than Friends of the Children, the After School Project funded intermediaries whose task was to organize the disparate groups and programs focused on after-school activities into a more coherent and durable system.

Before delving into the details of these initiatives, it is worth stepping back and taking a look at how a foundation dedicated to improving health and health care came to connect its mission to community-based programs working to give poor kids a chance to swing a bat in Little League, make pancakes in cooking classes, and spend an afternoon feeding animals at the petting zoo.

A New Take on Children's Health

The field of positive youth development sits under a very big tent. Its fundamental tenet—that children need guidance and support to grow into healthy adults—touches just about every unit of society: families, schools, police and other municipal services, and numerous social welfare agencies.

Also involved is a wide array of community and specialized organizations, including acknowledged pillars in the youth service field such as Big Brothers, Big Sisters, the Police Activities League, 4-H, and scouting. But experts believe that even organizations as esteemed as these can improve their programs—especially for disadvantaged children—by incorporating findings on youth development research.[4] The conviction rests mostly on theory; how to prove effectiveness continues to challenge the field.[5] Long-range measures include the usual benchmarks of success with at-risk youth: improved high school graduation rates, fewer teen pregnancies, and reduced juvenile substance abuse and crime. A few studies have run long enough to demonstrate that helping disadvantaged children improve interpersonal skills and emotional control during elementary school results in better academic performance and a smoother transition to adulthood.[6] But because the research is still new, virtually every strategy that flows from it provokes debate.

"Even among experts in the field—be they researchers or practitioners—there is no agreed-upon definition of positive youth development," Renée Wilson-Simmons, adolescent health expert and senior associate with the Annie E. Casey Foundation, writes in a comprehensive report on the field that was funded by the Robert Wood Johnson Foundation.[7] The closest thing to consensus, according to Wilson-Simmons, is "increasing clarity" about what children need for healthy development, including the following:

- Structured settings
- Physical and psychological safety
- Friends
- Positive relationships with adults who may also be role models
- Opportunities to build skills

In an ideal world, loving parents lay this groundwork for their children, exposing them to books, music, and educational toys, taking them to parks and museums, and inviting other children over to play. They have the maturity and the knowledge to leaven discipline with encouragement so youngsters can grow in competence and confidence. Good schools with dedicated teachers complement the work of such parents, creating a smooth path to adulthood. But how likely is such a scenario in today's world? Demographic studies show rising numbers of single-parent households, and even in two-parent households the norm today is two working parents. The result is an estimated five to fifteen million children in the United States who return from school to homes with no adult supervision for extended periods of time, according to the federal Department of Education.[8]

"We have to acknowledge that family structure is changing," says Floyd Morris, a former senior program officer at the Robert Wood Johnson Foundation, who helped develop its youth intervention portfolio. This structural change in families has led to exponential growth in afterschool programs, daycare, and other substitutes for the ideal world just sketched. "It goes to the issue of how do we care for our kids in the twenty-first century, and how do we transfer our values to the next generation," Morris says.

The Foundation's initial interest in positive youth development theory stemmed from concern about the toll on adolescents from accidental injury, pregnancy, and substance abuse, as well as corollaries to these behavioral health risks of school failure and underemployment. Studies also showed that substance abuse in the teenage years that leads to addiction often is a precursor to criminal activity, according to Kristin Schubert, a program officer at the Foundation, who supervises several youth intervention experiments.

Morris—who now heads Children's Futures, a Robert Wood Johnson Foundation-funded program that is working to improve infant and toddler health in Trenton, New Jersey—recalls growing interest at the Foundation in getting services to children before they succumbed to alcohol or drug addition or fell so far behind in school that dropping out seemed their only option. "We were looking at various studies that had been done around preventing substance use, violence, and those kinds of issues. One of the pieces of information we kept coming across was this notion that children who were disadvantaged were disconnected from a sufficient number of adults who could guide them through difficult passages and help them make the right choices."

A number of Foundation initiatives have incorporated this emerging research:

- A $14 million program called Free to Grow, which ran from 1992 to 2006, aimed at improving conditions in neighborhoods and strengthening the families of Head Start preschoolers so they might build the resilience necessary to steer clear of drugs and alcohol in their teen years.[9]
- The Urban Health Initiative (1995–2006, $60 million) sought to have a measurable impact on children's health in five cities by reducing substance abuse, smoking, street and domestic violence, teen pregnancy, infant mortality, and sexually transmitted disease. Mentoring and after-school programs were common threads in the projects undertaken in the five cities.[10]
- Reclaiming Futures (1999–2011, $27 million) focuses on young people who are already in trouble with alcohol or drugs—and the law. The program seeks to coordinate efforts by the juvenile justice system—police, juvenile courts, detention centers—and community-based treatment and support programs to comprehensively address the needs of substance-abusing youthful offenders.

- Best Friends (1990–2003, $2.18 million) worked with girls in grades six through twelve to discourage them from premarital intercourse, smoking, drinking, and drug abuse. The program also had a mentoring component: participating students were asked to choose a female teacher with whom they could talk about personal matters.[11]
- The Experience Corps (2001–2007, $6.8 million), which the Foundation helped to expand from five to nineteen participating cities, was devoted exclusively to mentoring. The program paired elementary school children with volunteer senior citizen mentors. The idea was to harness the talent and experience of older Americans who also had sufficient time to work one-on-one with children in need of both academic and social or emotional support. Experience Corps volunteers also worked closely with school officials and parents to develop before- and after-school enrichment programs. Those who contributed at least fifteen hours a week received a stipend of $100 to $200 a month, depending on the locale.

The Experience Corps was the Foundation's first experiment with monetary incentives provided to volunteer mentors. It paved the way for the Foundation's investment in Friends of the Children, a mentoring program that uses salaried, full-time professional mentors who are assigned to children for the duration of their school years. Foundation senior program officer Judith Stavisky says the model interested Foundation staff members because of its unusual approach toward positive youth development and its early track record of success in helping disadvantaged children to succeed in school and stay away from crime, alcohol, drugs, early parenting, and other threats during the volatile adolescent years. "The single most important factor that fosters resiliency in children is a consistent, long-term relationship with an adult," Stavisky says. "By paying someone a salary comparable to school teachers in a community, you attract individuals who are willing to commit to a position that provides both satisfaction and an income."

Friends of the Children

Duncan Campbell, sixty-three, strolls into the lobby of the Harvard Club on 43rd Street in New York City with the rolling gait of an athlete with creaky knees. In fact, Campbell worked his knees hard as a youth growing up in Portland, Oregon, competing for a berth in every sport he could squeeze into his high school schedule, then playing for YMCA and Boys Club teams in the evening. It was Campbell's way of avoiding the scene at home: his parents drunk to the point of incoherence, the house reeking of cigarette smoke and booze.

Campbell is at the Harvard Club to talk about the youth services program he founded called Friends of the Children. The setting for this conversation is as improbable as the stage Michael Oher now occupies at the University of Mississippi as one of pro football's hottest prospects. Campbell says his earliest memories are of long nights in taverns, wandering among the patrons while his parents tossed back drinks until closing time. Later, when the Oregon legislature barred minors from taverns, he stayed in the family car until his parents were ready to go home. A successful entrepreneur today, Campbell says he nevertheless remembers the fear and loneliness of his early years, his envy of children whose moms smiled and made dinner, and, most of all, his yearning for someone to talk to.

"There were police and bill collectors at the house all the time; my father was sent to prison twice," Campbell recalls. "We didn't ever have a conversation. I think we went to the beach once. I used to have to take care of him at night. He'd be drunk and say, 'Oh, you'll understand when you get older.'"

In time, Campbell did understand, but not in the way his father implied. The memories of his childhood led, he says, to a personal vow: to change at least one child's life "in reality, not just talk about it."

The result is Friends of the Children, an innovative mentoring program now being replicated nationally with support from the Robert Wood Johnson Foundation. Based in Portland, Oregon, Friends currently has chapters in Boston; Cincinnati; King County (Seattle), Washington; Klamath Falls, Oregon; New York City; and San Francisco. A two-and-half-year,

$1 million grant authorized by the Foundation in July 2005 and running through January 2008 is helping the program strengthen national oversight and quality control, and explore ways to reduce costs per child, currently averaging $9,000 annually.

The cost issue arises from the program's most noteworthy aspect: the use of highly trained mentors who commit to their assigned children for up to twelve years and earn salaries comparable to teachers' or social workers' in the local community. The experience so far, according to program officials, is that mentors average four to six years in the job. Hiring is selective and training is rigorous. Mentors are supervised and supported in their challenging and somewhat solitary work through weekly staff workshops and educational forums.

Mentors generally have eight children assigned to them. There are also shared activities among mentors so that when a mentor leaves the program, his or her children are reassigned to another mentor already familiar with the child. This ensures that children have a mentor until they graduate from high school. Job requirements include spending at least four hours a week with each child, helping him or her work toward grade-level academic performance, and compiling enriching and challenging experiences in line with the child's interests. Children are selected for participation in Friends in kindergarten or first grade, with parental approval. Getting children involved early in their schooling reflects the program's core tenet that academic success and attendant emotional and psychic rewards—self-confidence, goal development, hope for the future—are critical to disadvantaged children's long-term prospects. The program has performance goals, but they are set to be within reach of the youngsters selected for participation. Intermediate goals include:

- Improved social behavior and emotional control, and progress toward positive relationships with adults, peers, and community
- No substance abuse
- Academic progress, including improvements in attendance, classroom behavior, and reading, math, and computer proficiency
- Appropriate health care, both physical and mental

Overall goals for children graduating from the program are:

- High school diploma (preferred) or GED
- No involvement in the juvenile justice system
- No early parenting

Selecting children for participation in Friends is a rigorous process—and not for the softhearted. Indeed, the program hews closely to the research literature on resilience, looking to invest in children with innate tools to turn their lives around. Campbell shorthands the methodology by describing the target group as kindergartners testing between 17 and 31 on standardized tests with a hypothetical scale of 100. The reasoning is this: those scoring above 31 already are succeeding; those below 17 have too many learning and social deficits to benefit from Friends, and also are likely to be picked up by school-funded special education programs. The children Friends looks for have the potential to achieve in spite of severely handicapping backgrounds. Friends hopes to get them to 60; some have soared to 90.

The methodology of selection hews closely to the research on resiliency, according to Catherine Beckett, Friends' national program director. Each candidate undergoes up to six weeks of evaluation in partnership with school officials to determine both the "risk factors" confronting the child (including poverty, homelessness, domestic violence, or substance abuse in the home, to name a few) as well as the child's capacity in the form of "protective factors" (including high IQ, strong relational skills, extended family support, and so on) to meet program goals. Because success rests so heavily on the bond between mentor and child, children with conditions that hinder the development of relationships are not accepted, according to Beckett. These conditions include autism, psychosis, fetal alcohol syndrome, mental retardation (IQ below 75), and attachment disorders.

Results from Portland, where the program has the longest track record, are impressive. (Because other sites started later and are still several years from graduating their first class, this discussion focuses on the experience of Friends' Portland chapter, which has been in operation since 1993.) Of 272 boys and girls participating in Friends' Portland chapter in the 2005–2006 school year, 92 percent steered clear of the juvenile justice system and only one became pregnant (61 percent of the children in Friends' Portland chapter were born of teenage mothers). In 2006, thirty-six of forty-two students participating in the Friends program received high school diplomas or GEDs, and fourteen are pursuing college. In total, sixty-six young people have graduated from the Friends program. Eighty percent have graduated from high school or earned a GED; 68 percent were the first in their families to do so, and 40 percent have continued on to postgraduate education.

School officials in Portland testify to turnarounds in youngsters from tough backgrounds. The children—all poor, some from homes with troubled or non-English-speaking parents, others from no home at all but shifting between relatives and foster parents—typically arrive in kindergarten unprepared to sit still, take direction, and get along with peers. The attention they need is more than teachers can give in the classroom, resulting in school and social failure and unrealized potential.

"I remember one boy, a second-grader, sent to my office repeatedly who was so hostile—literally snarling," recalls John Horn, an area director for Portland Public Schools and former principal of Portland's Kelly Elementary School, where about 80 percent of the children are poor enough to qualify for the federal school lunch program. "This boy got assigned to a Friend, and I just watched him open up, learn how to handle situations, learn how to manage himself. It was amazing."

Getting some of these children to open up requires dogged resolve, mentors report. The job can be emotionally taxing—a major reason that Friends are paid professionals as opposed to volunteers, the customary workforce in mentoring programs.

"We had one child who wouldn't even talk to his Friend for two years," says Friends' Beckett. "Now their relationship is amazing."

Joe Bergen, the program director for the Portland chapter of Friends, who has been a Friend to several youngsters, recalls one of the first boys he mentored. The child had been physically and emotionally abused by his alcoholic father, and by the time he reached school age already had a deep reservoir of rage and mistrust. "He was really good at soccer but he could never finish a soccer game, because he'd blow up over something and start a fight,"

Bergen says. "Eventually, he was kicked off every team; his inability to control his emotions was ruining any chance of playing the sport he loved."

"I kept saying, 'I believe in you, you can do this!' When you show a child interest and stick by them and don't walk away even when they're goading you, there is a spirit that takes root and becomes infectious," Bergen says. "This boy now is proving to himself that he can do it. He's in sixth grade and playing on a soccer team and managing to stay in the game. His home life is still difficult—the family was recently evicted—and he may never have the tools to go to college, but that doesn't mean the program hasn't made a difference in his life." The confidence this boy gained through success in soccer crossed over into his school performance, according to Bergen, so much so that he now reads at grade level and gets along better with classmates and teachers.

Rachael Langtry, thirty-three, one of the program's first Friends, remembers mistakes she made in her first years, trying to steer the children to her choices—what to eat, how to spend free time—rather than work toward their own. Now a Friends team leader and bolstered by an intensive training program, Langtry helps new mentors avoid similar mistakes—as well as burnout. Friends learn many painful details about their charges' home lives—conditions they can't change and are required to steer clear of. The Friends job description is more precise today than it was when Langtry signed on thirteen years ago. It is to be a steadfast friend, as well as a guide to a larger world than most children in the program would otherwise know. Visits to the public library are a staple activity. So are field trips, hikes, cookouts with other Friends, and educational excursions as mundane as riding the public transit system so the children can learn how to get places safely on their own.

"The job is to walk alongside the child, be consistent, show up—this is really key for these kids," Langtry says.

So it was for Briita Vincent, one of Langtry's first assignments, now a biology major at Portland State University. "I was very shy when I was little," says Vincent, a composed, dark-eyed young woman of twenty. "School terrified me, and I cried all the time. I didn't know how to interact with other kids. Sometimes I'd lash out, sometimes I'd hide—literally under the desk."

The only child of a single mother with substance-abuse problems, Vincent says she was often lonely at home, and sought solace in books. "It was really good to have someone in my life like Rachael who could give me good advice. She was always very respectful in the way she communicated with me, and she was also a safe person, really careful about having me buckle up in the car, stuff like that."

Vincent's career goal is to be a zookeeper at the Oregon Zoo in Portland. She's paying for her education with a combination of federal Pell grants, a Friends of the Children scholarship, and earnings from two part-time jobs. She stays in touch with her mother by phone, but says they don't see each other much. Vincent laughs ruefully when asked how she came to be interested in animal care.

"Probably my upbringing," she deadpans. "Our house was really small—it had only one bedroom—and there was a period where we had twenty-seven cats and three dogs living with us."

Then she tackles the question in earnest: "When I was in eighth grade, I got into an internship program at the Portland zoo called Zoo Teen. Rachael told me about it. She knew I loved animals, and we were talking about what I could do over the summer. You had to apply for the internship, but I had no idea how to do that or what to say in an interview or anything. Rachael was really calm and encouraging about it. We practiced interview questions, and she got me to think about what teachers would give me a good recommendation. She got me to the interview, too."

"I loved that job," Vincent says. "We took care of the petting zoo animals and the pygmy goats in the Africa area. The petting zoo had ducks, bunnies, owls, lizards, and snakes, and we cleaned out their cages and made sure they had water and the right kind of food. That summer was the happiest time of my life."

The After School Project

The concept of scale is big in philanthropy today. Borrowed from economics and the high-tech field, scale in health and social philanthropy generally refers to experiments that have the potential to have an impact on a large number of people in a geographic region (compared with a small group of individuals in a demonstration project) or to be replicated in a great many sites throughout the country. It often refers to a program that could be picked up and funded by the government.

Testing the "scalability" of positive youth development theory was a driving force behind the Foundation's $16.9 million investment from 1999 to mid-2006 in After School: Connecting Children at Risk with Responsible Adults to Help Reduce Youth Substance Abuse and Other Health-Compromising Behaviors. Authorized as a demonstration project, After School set out to test whether the fractured landscape of urban programs covering out-of-school time could be organized around positive youth development principles so as to reduce youth substance abuse and other harmful behavior. The positive youth development goal that After School embraced was to connect disadvantaged youngsters with caring, responsible adults. But how to find these people, train them, and put them together with needy kids served by so many different programs?

"We saw this sort of multiheaded base of the schools, community organizations, city human services agencies, church-based and other kinds of programs serving kids," says Carol Glazer, a New York City–based management consultant who served as After School's national program director. "Then there was the continuum of small grassroots projects up to the big national franchise programs like the Boys Club and Big Brothers, Big Sisters. Then you add the parks departments, the libraries, and ultimately the police for children who have nothing else. . . ."

Designing the "scalability" mechanism was the central challenge, according to Glazer. To bring the program to a big enough scale, the Foundation's explicit charge to cities undertaking the experiment was to connect "more than 50 percent" of school children living in underserved urban neighborhoods with responsible adults in structured activities after school, on weekends, and during vacations. Unlike Friends of the Children, After School provided no direct services to children, nor did it control the staff of the programs where positive youth development theory was to be implemented. Its mission simply—or not so simply—was to get everyone armed with youth development research and marching in the same direction. In other words: communicate, listen, learn, convene, negotiate, train, and communicate some more. To accomplish this, After

School supported the development of coordinating infrastructures—the exact form differing from site to site—through which public and private youth organizations could learn how to enrich their programs, find collaborative partners in their field or neighborhood, and more efficiently reach at-risk school children. A specific goal of After School was to increase the participation in existing programs of youngsters from poor neighborhoods.

The Foundation selected three sites for comprehensive support: the San Francisco Bay Area, Chicago, and Boston. Two other sites, Milwaukee and San Jose, received limited technical assistance but no core funding.

The Bay Area's intermediary organization is called Team-Up for Youth. Serving San Francisco and Alameda counties, Team-Up helps to strengthen the quality of youth sports programs, with a goal of getting more low-income children to participate. Specifically, Team-Up provides grants and technical assistance to community-based sports organizations and offers training to foster a youth development focus in coaches and other staff. It also helps broker collaboration between public and private sector youth organizations; one effort, for example, led to a principal's opening up school space for a community-run summer sports program.

Chicago's intermediary organization is called After School Matters. It cultivates apprenticeship opportunities for high school students to enable them to work alongside professionals in arts, sports, technology, and communications. The program is structured as a public-private partnership and, in each participating neighborhood, involves a "community cluster" consisting of the local high school, public library and public recreational center. In addition to apprenticeships, After School Matters also organizes recreational clubs with appealing activities for public high school youths. The program increased the number of clusters from six to thirty-five and demonstrated that children who participated in apprenticeships or club activities had better school attendance.[12]

Boston's intermediary organization today is called Boston After-School & Beyond. Its history illustrates the time and effort needed to pull everyone under a single, conceptual tent. Only in 2004 was it possible to merge the Foundation-funded organization—originally called the Boston's After-School for All Partnership—with a preexisting effort by the city to address the needs of inner-city children, called the Mayor's 2:00-to-6:00 After-School Initiative. This finally created the public-private partnership necessary to pursue program goals, which are to expand after-school and summer opportunities in inner-city neighborhoods, improve the quality of programs citywide, and ensure adequate funding to support quality.

Many reports have been written about the After School Project, including an evaluation by Axiom Resource Management, Inc., of Falls Church, Virginia, which found the public-private partnership model to be an effective way to get the most out of existing resources, while also giving the After School project an avenue to influence public policy. And though building the organizational infrastructure in each city was a lengthy process that did not immediately yield measurable impact on youth, the evaluation concluded that this collaborative and evolutionary approach was likely to be more durable in the long run than if the After School sites were required to adhere to an inflexible design model.[13]

The goal here is not to duplicate these analyses, but to examine the difficulty of rescuing, en masse, children born into poverty. A tiny slice of the undertaking in Boston—bringing volunteer coaches on board with positive youth development theory—illustrates the complexity of achieving gains with disadvantaged youth on the scale of the After School Project.

The point man in Boston for the network of sports programs in Boston is Chris Lynch, a soft-spoken former elementary school teacher, and a coach and athlete in his own right. Lynch came to his current challenge from a more one-on-one experience with the potential of sports to help disadvantaged children build confidence and discipline, get healthy exercise, and improve school performance. In 1997, he began working at a youth development program in Boston called SquashBusters that a friend, Greg Zaff, had organized the previous year. His duties that first year weren't so different from a Friend's: mentoring, encouraging, and setting and enforcing standards of sportsmanship. Lynch recalls banging on doors in some of the city's toughest neighborhoods simply to make the point to one of his young players that skipping practice and letting down your teammates was not okay. From a pilot program with twenty-four middle school youngsters eager to whack a hard little ball around a four-walled court, SquashBusters today serves about three hundred children in

Boston and neighboring Cambridge, and it has inspired similar programs in New York City, Philadelphia, Chicago, Washington D.C., and San Diego.

However, Lynch's current job as head of the Boston Youth Sports Initiative—a division of Boston After School & Beyond—has exponentially more moving parts. No one even has an accurate count of all the sports programs in Boston. And the issues the project addresses go well beyond sports. Mariel Gonzales, Boston After School Beyond's chief operating officer, offers the example of a coalition partner who organized business leaders to create a work-study program for teenagers at risk for dropping out of school. Belatedly, they discovered that the children selected for the program lacked the social skills necessary to function in an office setting, leading to a proposal that Boston After School Beyond organize a remedial junior umpiring program so the teens could learn to mediate, communicate decisions, and handle authority. This potential solution was not orchestrated by the program's leaders so much as it was placed on the table for discussion in hopes that it would find a place on some organization's program agenda. "Everything we do is around network theory," says Lynch. "The idea is to get everyone to work together as a network to achieve their program's goals in the context of quality youth programming."

Lynch also is working on getting coaches—most of them volunteers—to undergo training in sports-based youth development, also called *character-based sports.* Along with teaching kids basic skills and how to win, this coaching model places emphasis on physical and emotional safety and age-appropriate instruction. In other words, a six-year-old T-baller should not be drilled like a varsity pitcher. But how much can you load on a volunteer coach? For the most part, these are people with jobs and families who, Lynch says, already have made "a huge commitment of personal time" to run practices, organize games, assemble equipment, arrange carpools, set schedules, communicate with parents, and handle innumerable other details. Lynch asks rhetorically, "Do we now require training as a condition for getting a sports league permit in order to foster positive youth development?"

Lynch's answer at this early stage of Boston After School's consensus-building effort is a resounding "No." The immediate effect, he believes, would be to drive some leagues out of business—no boon to the children now participating. Instead, Lynch is exploring a joint venture with Boston University's Institute for Athletic Coach Education whereby interested coaches might be sponsored for training so they, in turn, can pass the lessons on to fellow coaches.

"The issue is scale and intensity of training," Lynch says. "At the moment, everyone's doing things differently and everyone's reinventing the wheel. Moving beyond that is a long-term effort. We're still in the stage of finding out what's out there in terms of resources."

Conclusion

The plight of disadvantaged children has long been a rallying cry for social reformers. The novelist Charles Dickens wrote *Oliver Twist* in 1837 in part to lay bare the hypocrisy of England's 1834 Poor Law, which consigned those who couldn't support themselves to workhouses and, under the guise of social charity, brutally exploited their children for cheap labor. In this century, advocates for children orphaned by the unchecked spread of AIDS in sub-Saharan Africa have helped galvanize international medical relief efforts.

In the United States, well-established and popular government aid programs for disadvantaged children include family- and school-based nutrition supplements (WIC, food stamps, and school breakfast and lunch programs) and health care services through Medicaid and the State Children's Health Insurance Program. At the community level, many people participate as organizers, volunteers, and benefactors to sustain activities for local youth, including sports, art, music, tutoring, scouting, community service, and mentoring. Such grassroots efforts are complemented by established national programs, including scouts, Little League, Boys and Girls Clubs, and YMCAs.

Philanthropic organizations like the Robert Wood Johnson Foundation also are in the mix. They help sustain programs of proven value while supporting experiments like After School and Friends of the Children with the potential to be tomorrow's mainstays. An early initiative of the Foundation, for example, tested the feasibility of locating primary care clinics in schools serving children with no other source of medical care.[14]

Twenty-five years later, school-based clinics have become commonplace. More recent investments by the Foundation in mentoring programs recognize disadvantaged children's emotional and psychological needs. The mentoring programs are grounded in the emerging science of human resiliency, which focuses on innate as well as external factors—called "protective"—that help people navigate adversity. The research is exciting to counselors, teachers, social workers, and others who work with children because it delineates a sturdier framework for rescuing disadvantaged youngsters than the intuitive good will behind so many ad hoc efforts. It also offers a new direction for policy—from one focused on remedying children's weaknesses to one that builds on their strengths. Hence, the titular umbrella under which advocates have organized: positive youth development.

But the field is still new. There are few long-term studies to document cause-and-effect changes in the trajectory of children's lives from either sustained, one-on-one interventions like Friends of the Children or broad community embrace of positive youth development theory as in After School. A handful of studies have looked at young adults who at some point in their school years participated in programs to help them steer clear of substance abuse and crime. None of these efforts comes close to the intensity of Friends of the Children; many are in-class or pull-out programs to help children build interpersonal and self-management skills. Some specifically aim to reduce substance abuse and crime in the teenage years through this type of emotional and psychological skill building. One such program is the Seattle Social Development Project, which works with children in eighteen public elementary schools in various neighborhoods of Seattle. Through interviews with participants who had reached age twenty-one, researchers found that the program had significant positive effects on school and work performance and mental health, but less impact on crime and substance abuse.[15]

There's also a dearth of information on which children are most likely to benefit, and no consensus on what constitutes success. The current measures—high school diploma and avoidance of crime and substance abuse—reflect traditional child welfare goals of reducing personal and social harm. However, those using resilience theory on a day-to-day basis—

for example, the mentor cadre at Friends of the Children and After School's community outreach workers—emphasize subtler benchmarks of success such as self-confidence and self-respect, the ability to make and keep friends, and the capacity to trust others. Their comments call to mind the boy in Portland who learned to get through a soccer game without fighting—and only then began to get along and perform better in school. The path to this much-desired self-mastery remains more easily described by anecdote than science and provides evidence of the work still ahead for researchers. And as Wilson-Simmons notes, even positive youth development experts have trouble agreeing on a common definition of their field.

The Foundation's investments in Friends of the Children and After School are consistent with its history of support for health-related youth programs, all of which aim to assist children trapped by harsh and potentially harmful circumstances beyond their control. With Friends of the Children and After School, the Foundation explicitly challenged the programs, albeit in different ways, to demonstrate the applicability of positive youth development theory on a scale sufficient to improve many lives at an affordable price. In the case of Friends of the Children, that means bringing down the cost per child, currently $9,000 annually or more than $100,000 by the time a participant graduates from high school. In After School, the challenge was to get more than half of school-aged youngsters living in poor urban neighborhoods to participate in activities through which they could build relationships with responsible adults.

Neither program has explicitly met those challenges—nor do their leaders entirely agree that these are appropriate litmus tests for success. For After School, the task of getting public and private sector youth services organizations to talk to one another and embrace the idea of joint planning was bigger than anyone expected, and this delayed enrollment outreach, participants say. At Friends, the pressure of funders to reduce costs per child has led its founder, Duncan Campbell, to issue a challenge of his own. Campbell wants funders to consider what he calls the "business case" for "value" investments in high-risk children to prevent the costly consequences of failure—up to $60,000 a year for juvenile incarceration.[16]

The debate within and around Friends of the Children and After School underscores the important role of philanthropy in nurturing ideas with the potential to improve people's lives. At issue in these experiments was a largely untested social construct—resilience theory—in a new field called positive youth development that is still working to define itself. Intuitively, the emphasis on reaching children early in their schooling and playing to their strengths makes sense. But the logistics of doing that are tougher than anticipated—highlighting the need for more studies asking a broader range of questions to truly bring the field of positive youth development to scale.

Notes

1. Lewis, M. "The Ballad of Big Mike." *New York Times Magazine,* Sept. 24, 2006.
2. Zimmerman, P. Building Intensive Relationships with At-Risk Children: The Research and Literature at a Glance. Report funded by the Children's Institute of Oregon.
3. The Robert Wood Johnson Foundation Grants Results Report. Youth Development Programs Hold Promise, Often Fall Short, 2003. (http://www.rwjf.org/portfolios/resources/grantsreport.jsp?filename=035504.htm&iaid=131&gsa=5).
4. Roth, J. L., and others. "Promoting Healthy Adolescence: Synthesis of Youth Development Program Evaluations." *Journal of Research on Adolescence,* 1998, *8,* 423–459.
5. Durlak, J. A., and Weissberg, R. P. *The Impact of After-School Programs that Promote Personal and Social Skills.* Chicago: Collaborative for Academic, Social, and Emotional Learning (CASEL), 2007.
6. Hawkins, J. D., and others. "Promoting Positive Adult Function Through Social Development Intervention in Childhood: Long-Term Effects from the Seattle Social Development Project." *Archives of Pediatric Adolescent Medicine,* 2005, *159*(5), 469.
7. Wilson-Simmons, R. "Positive Youth Development: an Examination of the Field." Prepared for the Robert Wood Johnson Foundation, May 2006, 6. (http://www.rwjf.org/files/publications/other/PYDTopicSummary.pdf?gsa=1).
8. U.S. Department of Education: After School Programs: Keeping Children Safe and Smart. 2000 (http://www.ed.gov/pubs/afterschool/index.html).
9. Wielawski, I. "Free to Grow." *To Improve Health and Health Care, Vol. IX: The Robert Wood Johnson Foundation Anthology.* San Francisco: Jossey-Bass, 2006.
10. See Chapter Seven in this volume.
11. See Chapter Three in this volume.

12. Conwal Division of Axiom Resource Management, Inc. Final Evaluation Report of the After School Project, 2006.
13. Ibid. See also Proscio, T. "Making the Most of the Day: the Final Report of the After School Project," 2006. (www.theafterschoolproject.org/RepoProg-list0.html).
14. Wielawski, I. "The Local Initiative Funding Partners Program." *To Improve Health and Health Care 2000: The Robert Wood Johnson Foundation Anthology.* San Francisco: Jossey-Bass, 2000.
15. Hawkins and others, 2005.
16. Tyler, J. L., Zeidenberg, J., and Lotke, E. *Cost-Effective Corrections: The Fiscal Architecture of Rational Justice Systems.* Washington, D.C.: The Justice Policy Institute, 2006.

CHAPTER 9

The Robert Wood Johnson Foundation's Approach to Evaluation

James R. Knickman and Kelly A. Hunt

Editors' Introduction

Foundations, as Michael Porter and Mark Kramer observed in an influential article published in 1999, are often ambivalent about evaluation. "The overall failure to evaluate the results of foundation grants is the most telling danger sign of all. Almost no money is set aside for program evaluation . . . [yet] without evaluation, a foundation will never know whether or not it has been successful."[1] Evaluation has become more important in the field of philanthropy since then, however, as foundation boards and staff members increasingly demand evidence of the impact of their grantmaking and as policymakers and the public insist on more accountability.

The Robert Wood Johnson Foundation has placed a high priority on program evaluation since its inception as a national philanthropy in 1972. It has developed a four-tiered system of evaluation that ranges from the evaluation of individual grants and clusters of grants to the qualitative assessments found in *The Robert Wood Johnson Foundation Anthology* series.

In this chapter, two architects of the Foundation's evaluation system describe that system and examine its strengths and weaknesses. As the Foundation's vice president for research and evaluation between 1992 and 2006, James R. Knickman was the person primarily responsible for the Foundation's approach to evaluation. Kelly A. Hunt, who was at the Foundation between 2000 and 2006, was a research officer and in charge of the Foundation's "scorecard." Knickman is currently the president and chief executive officer of the New York State Health Foundation, and Hunt is a senior program director there.

This is the first comprehensive public presentation of the way that the Robert Wood Johnson Foundation assesses its programs and their effectiveness. As such, it may resonate with other foundations and nonprofit organizations seeking to have a better understanding of the impact of their activities.

Notes

1. Porter, M. E., and Kramer, M. R. "Philanthropy's New Agenda: Creating Value." *Harvard Business Review,* Nov.–Dec. 1999, 121–130.

In philanthropy, as in business, the bottom line counts. But each sector measures the bottom line differently. Businesses can look to revenue, income, sales, earnings per share, and other quantitative indicators to measure performance. Foundations often work with less clear-cut indicators of impact. Sometimes they find it difficult to quantify the objective they wish to achieve. At other times it is difficult to know whether social change is due to the actions of a foundation or to other forces.

Over the past twenty years, the imperative to evaluate outcomes and assess effectiveness has become progressively important in philanthropy. Government leaders and others who watch philanthropy increasingly push for evidence that foundations use their resources wisely and actually contribute to addressing social problems. Boards of trustees at foundations have also become increasingly demanding when it comes to accountability and impact.

This imperative for evaluation is most characteristic among foundations that attempt to effect social change in active, coordinated ways. If a foundation chooses to focus on direct charity—funding services at homeless shelters, say, or supporting free medical care for the uninsured—the links between social contributions and the foundation's resources are generally considered self-evident. The impact of such contributions can be measured by the number of people served or by improvement in their health. When a foundation focuses on making grants that address a social problem, such as efforts to end homelessness or to bring about universal health insurance coverage, then it becomes more difficult to demonstrate a causal relationship between a foundation's investment and a change in the social environment.

The Robert Wood Johnson Foundation is generally regarded as a foundation that takes evaluation and performance assessment seriously. It has a staff of twelve professionals plus support staff members focused on evaluation, and it has been conducting evaluations of grants since its earliest days, in the 1970s.

Historical Roots

The idea of evaluating the effectiveness of grant programs came naturally to the early leaders of the Foundation. The board of directors consisted largely of recently retired Johnson & Johnson executives and others who had been colleagues of the founder. Accustomed to drug trials in which the effectiveness of a new pharmaceutical product is rigorously tested before being placed on the market, the board looked for comparable approaches to judging the impact of Foundation programs. Many of the Foundation's earliest investments were multisite demonstrations of new approaches to improving access to health care. Multiple states or communities or providers would be funded to try a specified strategy for, say, improving access. This type of grantmaking warranted investments in program evaluations to determine whether or not the new approach in fact had beneficial impacts. Given the interest of the Foundation in identifying ideas that could, if successful, serve as models, evaluation emerged as a central feature of its approach to grantmaking over the years.

Additionally, the 1970s, when the field of public policy analysis was emerging, were years of ferment in the area of social science research. It was natural to borrow the evaluation methods being used by the federal government to test new approaches to delivering services to low-income individuals ("social experiments"). In the 1970s, for example, the federal government financed a range of social experiments that tested new ideas in welfare reform, national health insurance models, and workforce training.

The emphasis on formal evaluations of large-scale programs continued through the 1980s, and it continues today for programs that test new ideas for improving health care or promoting the public's health. During the 1980s and 1990s, however, the Foundation's grantmaking approaches became more diversified as it funded research to understand health challenges such as the lack of insurance coverage; communications efforts to increase public awareness about a range of health problems and potential solutions to them; and wide-ranging programs to address health problems such as smoking. The board also applied pressure to broaden the approaches used by the Foundation to assess impact. Board members asked two types of questions: What are we learning from all of these grants? and

How can we be sure that our grants are really making a difference in improving health or health care?

As a result, in the 1990s evaluation at the Foundation began to change in important ways. Instead of just asking whether a specific grant program was effective, the Foundation began looking at groups of grants that were meant to affect a specific health problem and assessing whether the grants as a group were effective in addressing it. It developed a family of evaluation tools focused on different aspects of impact. The Foundation currently uses a four-tiered approach to evaluation.

- The first tier attempts to understand the effectiveness of specific programs. Following its well-established pattern, the Foundation hires outside institutions to evaluate the results of its major grant initiatives.
- The second tier attempts to understand the impact of clusters of programs that focus on a particular goal or set of goals. In 2003, the Foundation developed an impact framework that sets short-, long-, and medium-range targets in specific program areas (such as health insurance coverage, childhood obesity, and public health).[1] Concurrently, it developed performance indicators to measure progress toward those targets.
- The third tier examines how the Foundation as an organization is doing, using a "scorecard" that is presented to the board annually. The scorecard incorporates the impact framework's performance indicators and commissions surveys to find out what grantees think of the Foundation, what experts think the Foundation's impact on health is, and what the staff considers to be the Foundation's strong and weak points.
- The fourth tier assesses the work of the Foundation in a less formal way and presents the results to a broad public. This collaborative program-evaluation-communications effort uses two vehicles: (1) grant results reports, in which the Foundation commissions writers to investigate specific grants and grant programs and write reports on them that appear on

the Foundation's Web site, and (2) *To Improve Health and Health Care: The Robert Wood Johnson Foundation Anthology,* the book series published annually by Jossey-Bass. Both of these vehicles focus on disseminating what the Foundation has learned from various aspects of its grantmaking.

Tier 1: Measuring the Impact of Specific Programs

If a state government requires schools to report to parents on their child's body mass index, will it result in lower rates of childhood obesity over time? If frail elders are given an option to hire their adult children or neighbors as caregivers instead of requiring the elders to use formal long-term care workers, will outcomes improve and costs decrease? If a hospital provides readily accessible translation services for non-English-speaking patients, will they become healthier?

These are the types of questions that can be answered through carefully designed program evaluations. For many years, the Foundation has funded independent researchers at universities and other organizations to conduct studies that assess whether the interventions it has funded improve outcomes. It is not coincidental that the Foundation relies on outside evaluators. Having an external, independent team measuring outcomes keeps the process honest. It is too easy for a foundation's program staff and its grantees to become overinvested in a program and reluctant to admit that they have not achieved the desired result. Moreover, when an intervention is successful, the judgment of an independent team increases the credibility of evaluation findings.

Program evaluations also look at implementation issues to learn why outcomes are reached or not and to document how a grantee goes about working on an initiative. Implementation analyses sometimes can help grantees midstream, and most important, they create a roadmap of do's and don'ts that can help in the replication of successful programs.

Program evaluations funded by the Robert Wood Johnson Foundation generally use social science and epidemiological research design concepts. At the heart of this tier of evaluation is comparison: whenever possible, the evaluation team compares outcomes at sites supported by the Foundation with those at similar sites not supported by the Foundation. In the ideal program evaluation, either random assignment or some other mechanism is used to ensure that the comparison sites are as similar as possible to the Foundation-supported sites.

Over the years, the Foundation has learned how difficult it is to mount evaluations in the real world. The perfect evaluation design is generally elusive, baseline data may not be available, and second-best strategies for selecting comparison groups and measuring outcomes are often necessary. Even with the best of intentions, programs tend to evolve over time as priorities change, expected outcomes are revised, or grantees shift their focus. Tensions between program staff and evaluation team members can complicate the evaluation process, and the burden on grantees and program staff members to meet the needs of evaluators is frequently greater than was projected at the start. Often, the findings that emerge are inconclusive or are reported too late to influence decisions about next steps in the Foundation's grantmaking or to inform public opinion.

Thus, the practical difficulties in carrying out rigorous program evaluations are enormous. The evaluation of the Fighting Back program, a nearly $100 million initiative to foster community coalitions to reduce substance abuse in high-risk neighborhoods, provides a classic case study. The program changed course in midstream; the evaluation began after the program was halfway through; the composition of the communities changed; the program office and the evaluation team could not agree on the indicators to be measured; and when the evaluation was finally completed, its findings were strongly disputed.[2]

Whatever the practical difficulties, evaluations do result in learning. Both the Foundation and those outside it use the results of evaluation to develop programs. SUPPORT and Cash & Counseling offer two examples of the practical use of evaluations.

SUPPORT—the Study to Understand Prognoses and Preferences for Outcomes and Risks of Treatments—tested new approaches to providing care for terminally ill hospitalized patients; it involved patients, their families, nurses, and physicians in determining the kind of care that the patients would receive toward the end of their lives. As the demonstration project was being carried out in five hospitals, there was a sense among those involved in it that patients and their families were in fact making better choices, and that their wishes were being respected more. When the research findings were tabulated, however, clear evidence emerged that patients' wishes were not respected and that their care was no different from that of patients who did not receive the special intervention. These findings led to a fundamental rethinking of end-of-life care and paved the way for a decade of Foundation-funded initiatives to reshape the care of terminally ill patients.

The evaluation of the Cash & Counseling program compared the satisfaction levels of people receiving long-term care services from home health care agencies supported by Medicaid to those of another group that was given the option of using family, friends, or community members to deliver the services. The findings of the evaluation demonstrated much higher satisfaction rates among the people given the new option. Timing and reliability of care, treatment of beneficiaries by caregivers, and performance of tasks by caregivers were also substantially better for this group. The evaluation findings provided a basis for recent legislation that expands the Cash & Counseling approach from a three-state demonstration project to an option available in all fifty states.

Evaluations suggesting that no impact was associated with an initiative have led the Foundation to shift priorities. For example, when an evaluation concluded that a fellowship program to improve the understanding and teaching of health care financing was ineffective, the Foundation decided to discontinue the program.[3] Similarly, a negative evaluation of a program to encourage community partnerships to lower the cost of health insurance led the Foundation to end the program and reassess the approach.[4]

The Foundation's long experience in program evaluation has led to numerous lessons, among them:

- It is essential to design programs and evaluations at the same time so that a program can be implemented in a manner that makes an evaluation feasible.
- It is also essential to get timely baseline data if before-and-after comparisons are a feature of an evaluation.

- Evaluation findings need to emerge in a timely manner. Great insights that arrive too late to influence the next steps or federal or state policy have no impact.
- Evaluation design needs to be flexible enough to adjust to changing features of the program being evaluated. Few programs are implemented as planned, and most end up being less ambitious in scope than originally projected.
- The evaluation team and the program team need to work together. Whenever tension, a lack of respect, or an inability to work together characterizes a demonstration initiative, it is unusual for useful findings to emerge.
- Evaluations tend to be stronger when a program has clearly defined and clearly measurable expected outcomes.

Tier 2: Performance Indicators: Tracking the Impact of a Portfolio of Programs

Although program evaluations can measure the success or failure of individual programs, the Foundation's trustees and staff want to know what impact its grantmaking *in a specific field* is having. For example, when the Foundation sets an objective such as reducing tobacco use, they want to know whether smoking has gone down and, to the extent it is possible to know, what contribution the Foundation's programs have made to the decline.

Grantmaking at the Robert Wood Johnson Foundation is mainly directed at attempting to achieve tangible improvement in some aspect of the health system or health-related behavior. The staff and the trustees identify a behavior or public health, health care system, or policy issue that is of concern—such as tobacco use, childhood obesity, or the rising number of uninsured persons—agree upon a specific strategic objective (such as lowering the number of uninsured people by a certain percentage within a specified time period), and then decide on an array of grants that they expect will meet the strategic objective.

To assess whether progress is being made, staff members set down a series of performance indicators that must be reached for the strategic objective to be achieved. These performance indicators are used by the board and the senior staff to judge performance and to guide decisions about resource allocation. Objectives are modified from time to time—often in three- to five-year intervals—but sometimes a priority remains in place for ten or more years.

The performance indicators flow from logic models that the staff develops. These specify, in simple terms, what has to happen in the short- and mid-term and then the intermediate term if the Foundation can expect to achieve a specified objective in the long run. Short-term indicators are meant to be roughly annual checks on progress that help clarify the Foundation's immediate plans and strategies. A short-term indicator for the tobacco-reduction goal might be convening a summit meeting to help frame policy priorities, followed up by a coordinated plan of action developed by grantees working in this field. Intermediate indicators are measures—often more ambitious than short-term performance indicators—that the Foundation uses to determine progress over a two- to three-year time period. As one example, the Foundation looked at the proportion of the population covered by clean indoor air laws as an intermediate indicator of progress toward its goal of reducing smoking. Long-term indicators reach beyond three years and are broader in focus and level of impact. In the area of tobacco, the Foundation tracked the prevalence of youth smoking as a long-term indicator. Table 9.1 presents a performance indicator report—with short-, medium-, and long-term indicators—that the Foundation staff and board used to track progress in tobacco control.

Each performance indicator—whether short-, intermediate-, or long-term—is also assigned a level of control or influence that indicates how much effect the staff thinks the Foundation can have on reaching it. For example, it is well within the control of the Foundation to organize a meeting of experts on national health insurance, so it would be given a "high" level of control; reducing the number of uninsured by, say, 50 percent depends on factors beyond the Foundation's control and would thus be given a "low" level of control.

Developing this performance assessment system was a major undertaking for the staff. Each internal Foundation team assigned to a specific area of grantmaking was asked to specify the concrete objectives it sought to achieve (such as reducing tobacco use by children, improving retention of nurses, or reducing the disparities among racial or ethnic groups in the care they receive for cardiac conditions). The outcome specified by the objective

Table 9.1. Strategic Indicators: Tobacco

Tracking Indicators

Indicators	**Control**	**Target Date**	**Baseline Status**	**Current Status**	**Target**
State tobacco control funding as a percentage of the CDC minimum (tracking backslide)	M	7/08	40.2% (2000)	22.1% (as of 12/05)	27.0%
Prevalence of cigarette use among 12th graders (tracking backslide)	L	7/08	31.4% (2000)	23.2% (as of 12/05)	25.0%
"Strength of Tobacco Control" Index-monitors tobacco control capacity at state level (tracking backslide)	M	7/08	0 (Normalized/ 2000	2.4 (as of 12/04)	2.4
Short-term Indicators (4/1/05–4/1/06)	**Control**	**Target Date**	**Baseline Status**	**Current Status**	**Target**
Implemented fund-raising strategy with management	H	7/05	Not completed	Completed (7/05)	To complete
Completed transition plans and budgets for major programs	H	10/05	Not completed	Completed (10/05)	To complete
Intermediate Indicators (13–36 Months)	**Control**	**Target Date**	**Baseline Status**	**Current Status**	**Target**
Combined average state and federal tobacco excise tax	H	7/06	$1.11 (2003)	$1.33 (as of 9/06 Completed (10/05	$1.25
Proportion of the population covered by comprehensive clean indoor air laws	H	7/06	21.8% (2003)	33.1% (+.09%, 6/06) Partially completed	35.0%
Number of states that cover tobacco dependence treatment through Medicaid (tracking backslide)	L	7/06	38 (2003)	41 (as of 12/05) Completed (12/05)	35
Long-term Indicators (+36 Months)	**Control**	**Target Date**	**Baseline Status**	**Current Status**	**Target**
Prevalence of youth cigarette use (high school students, grades 9–12)	L	7/07	28.5% (2001)	23.0% (+1.1%, 6/06) Completed (7/04)	23.0%

Table 9.1. Strategic Indicators: Tobacco, Cont'd.

Tracking Indicators

Long-term Indicators (+36 Months)	**Control**	**Target Date**	**Baseline Status**	**Current Status**	**Target**
Prevalence of adult cigarette use	L	7/07	23.2% (2000)	21.1% (+0.2%, early release data as of 6/06)	18.0%
Number of states dedicating CDC-recommended amounts of MSA/tax dollars for tobacco prevention/ control	L	7/08	4 (2003)	4 (as of 12/05)	10

Control: L = Low, M = Medium, H = High

Source: Report to the board of trustees of the Robert Wood Johnson Foundation, October 2006.

had to be measurable so that the Foundation's board and the senior staff would know whether the Foundation's grantmaking had had an impact.

The performance measures serve as signposts that help the staff and the board assess whether or not positive change is likely to occur over the long term. If short- and medium-term targets are not met, then the long-term objectives are unlikely to be met as well. The assessment of short- and medium-term objectives can lead the Foundation to alter its strategy (and the logic model guiding it), increase the level of the intervention, or perhaps reconsider the feasibility of reaching the ultimate goal.

Performance measurement is difficult. It is challenging to identify tangible targets that can be measured and that can actually change in the short or intermediate run but do not seem trivial. In managing the process, there is constant concern that focusing on measurable outcomes could lead the Foundation to address less important, though more easily measurable, problems or to adopt less risky program strategies.

The Foundation uses the performance measurement system to force more systematic thinking and to present clear choices. It also forces the staff to concentrate on common, agreed-upon goals. Although the performance measurement system provides guidance for decision making and resource allocation, it is not followed slavishly. The board is sometimes willing to approve grant initiatives even knowing that it will prove difficult to measure the results of the Foundation's investment. For example, it is difficult to demonstrate concrete results of the Foundation's human capital portfolio, but the Foundation's staff and board believe that it is important. Of course, there are critics on both sides of the Foundation's approach to performance measurement. Some at the Foundation feel that the system drives out attention to important objectives that are difficult to quantify. Others feel that the Foundation still does not insist enough on measuring impact in some areas of its grantmaking.

Tier 3: The Scorecard: Assessing Organizational Effectiveness

The Foundation's annual scorecard has become an integral part of its self-assessment—a tool for senior management, the staff, and the board to assess how the Foundation is doing in a number of areas. It creates a time for formal reflection on the organization's performance and also provides staff members and trustees with a method of identifying and addressing weak areas of organizational performance. For more than a decade, the scorecard has represented an important tool for holding the Foundation accountable to its mission and its guiding principles.

In creating its balanced scorecard, the Foundation adapted a concept developed by the Harvard Business School professor Robert S. Kaplan and the businessman David P. Norton for measuring performance in the business world.[5] Typically, in the business sector these measurements include financial, internal business, innovation and learning, and customers. The Robert Wood Johnson Foundation, whose bottom line is social change rather than profitability, translated these measurements into program impact, program development, customer (that is, grantee) service, and human/financial capital. It also incorporates, as an appendix, a review of grants management performance.

Program Impact

The first section of the scorecard considers whether the Foundation is meeting the goals it set for itself, by presenting the performance indicators for each portfolio and program area. Performance indicators are summarized in terms of the percentage that were completed on time, late, partly completed, or not competed at all. Some commentary on the stability of the indicators is included here, too—whether small or even major changes were made to any indicators in a particular programming area. Although some amount of change to indicators is to be expected in order to maintain the flexibility to adapt to changes in the environment, a complete lack of stability could indicate a lack of sound programming at the beginning.

Also incorporated in the program impact section are data from external audiences: grantees and outside "thought leaders"—a group that includes heads of prominent health organizations, academics, public health officials, Medicaid officials, federal policymakers, state legislators, and the health media. The Foundation's grantees, who have a wide range of expertise, include health researchers, practitioners, advocates, decision makers, and executives. Their judgments about the Foundation's presence, priorities, and effectiveness are an important gauge for the Foundation. Grantees rate the Foundation's impact in a number of ways, including

- Impact on the field, advancement of knowledge in the field, and effect on public policy in grantees' fields
- Objectivity of programming and disseminated materials
- Skill and knowledge of staff
- Influence of programming and communications on health care leaders and policymakers

Thought leaders are asked similar questions, though they are also specifically asked to rate the Foundation's impact on particular programming areas, such as tobacco use, public health, and health insurance coverage. They are also asked to indicate their confidence in, and the usefulness of, information produced by the Foundation.

The grantee and thought leader survey allows the Foundation to compare itself to other foundations. The Center for Effective Philanthropy conducts the grantee survey and directs similar questions to grantees of the Robert Wood Johnson Foundation and other foundations. The Center can then let the Foundation know how it stacks up with other foundations. The thought leader survey asks respondents to rate the Robert

Wood Johnson Foundation with a set of its peers, including the Henry J. Kaiser Family Foundation, the W.K. Kellogg Foundation, the Commonwealth Fund, the Pew Charitable Trusts, the California HealthCare Foundation, and the California Endowment. In sum, this section of the scorecard provides the staff and the board with both internal and external indicators and assessments of the Foundation's impact.

Program Development

The scorecard's program development section examines the strength of the Foundation's programming efforts, such as the soundness of its strategies and whether its interests are in line with those of its grantees, thought leaders, and the public. For example, the program development section reviews whether the public perceives health care as a major priority for the government to address, as well as specific health concerns—such as cost, quality, and the uninsured—to get a sense of whether the public's and the Foundation's priorities are aligned. The reasons for including this information in program development are twofold. First, though Robert Wood Johnson is a private foundation, it considers itself to be accountable to the public interest. Second, information about public perceptions of important health topics—childhood obesity, for example—can help guide the Foundation's programming. Moreover, if a topic is of great concern to public health professionals but does not resonate with the public or policymakers, it is an opportunity for the Foundation to inform the public through its communications efforts.

The program development section also incorporates thought leaders' opinions of various health and health care priorities. In 2006, for example, over 90 percent of thought leaders thought that health insurance coverage was a high or very high priority for the nation.

Finally, information from both thought leaders and grantees helps the Foundation understand whether these constituents feel that it is

- Working on issues important to the United States
- Making long-term commitments to important issues
- Supporting and building leadership in health and health care

Customer Service

The survey of grantees, conducted by the Center for Effective Philanthropy, asks how they feel the Foundation is treating them (see box). Indicators from this survey form the basis of the customer service section of the scorecard and include questions such as these:

- Is the Foundation clear about the types of proposals it will fund?
- Is it clear in communicating its goals and objectives?
- Is it fair throughout the application process and responsive throughout the lifetime of a project?
- Are the Foundation's program officers approachable, courteous, and helpful?
- Is the technical assistance provided by or through the Foundation adequate?

The seriousness with which the Foundation takes this information is illustrated by its response to the grantee survey in 2004 that indicated its customer service was not up to that of other foundations. This led to an internal "quality improvement initiative" that resulted in an almost complete overhaul of the Foundation's grant review and approval procedures and the way in which staff members communicated with grantees and potential grantees.

Staff Satisfaction and Financial Performance

This section of the scorecard looks first within the Foundation to determine what the staff thinks of it as a place to work (see box). This includes information about the staff's overall satisfaction, its ratings of management, and opinion of its ability to communicate concerns up through the ranks of the Foundation.

This section of the scorecard also reports on how the investment portfolio is doing. The indicators include the return rate and the volatility of the Foundation's endowment portfolio.

The Grantee, Thought Leader, and Public Opinion Surveys

The *grantee survey* asks approximately three hundred grantees about key aspects of the Foundation's service, programs, and impact. It contains questions on

- Grantees' perceptions of the Foundation's impact on their organizations and their field
- Whether the Foundation is addressing the most important health and health care issues and is willing to commit the time and the resources needed to achieve its goals
- How fair the staff is in its interactions with grantees
- Whether the grant application and reporting requirements are burdensome
- How clearly the Foundation communicates its goals and strategies

The survey is confidential and allows for comparisons over time. Recently, it has allowed for comparisons with other funders because of the Foundation's participation in a survey fielded by the Center for Effective Philanthropy that elicits similar information from a number of foundations. Finally, the Foundation periodically surveys applicants it has turned down to look for warning signals coming from this group.

The *thought leader survey* interviews decision makers from universities, health plans, hospitals, health associations, government, the media, and public health organizations. Those in this group are questioned about their knowledge of the Robert Wood Johnson Foundation as an organization and their views on its priorities, its reputation, and the quality of the information it produces. Those who are familiar with the Foundation are asked to rate its impact in addressing problems related to health and health care as well as the impact of its specific strategic areas (for example, quality of care or health insurance coverage). This survey is also confidential, and it, too, allows for comparisons over time.

The *public opinion survey* queries the public about their views on the top issues facing the nation and the Foundation's priorities. Respondents are asked to list the issues they think the government should be addressing and to rate the American health care and public health systems. They are also asked to name the top medical care and public health concerns facing the nation. The survey then asks respondents to rank the Foundation's areas of interest and a few other select health care issues.

The *staff survey,* which is also confidential, asks staff members how well they think the Foundation is doing in meeting its guiding principles—a core set of values that promote good stewardship of Foundation resources, fairness in the treatment of grantees and the field, and professional, ethical staff conduct. The staff survey asks a number of questions to determine whether that staff members feel that the guiding principles are honored by the leadership of the Foundation and are useful in guiding everyday transactions. It also asks questions related to the working environment at the Foundation and the staff's judgment of the Foundation's program development and impact. For example, staff members are asked whether sufficient effort is made to get their opinions, whether there is an environment of teamwork at the Foundation, and whether the Foundation has clear goals and objectives.

Grants Management Performance

The scorecard also contains, as an appendix, a review of data from the Foundation's grants management system to see how many applications are being submitted and, ultimately, being funded; and how the work of the Foundation and its grantees is being disseminated in print and on the Web. It also contains a section that outlines changes that were and will be made.

Tier 4: Grant Results Reports and *The Robert Wood Johnson Foundation Anthology* Series

The fourth tier of the Robert Wood Johnson Foundation's evaluative activities, which identifies and shares lessons from the Foundation's grantmaking, takes the form of two publication vehicles: the grant results reports and the annual *Robert Wood Johnson Foundation Anthology.* Both take a broader view of evaluation and attempt to share the understanding gained from the Foundation's investments with as wide an audience as possible.

The grant results reports now total more than two thousand distinct reports that are posted on the Foundation's Web site. The reports are prepared by a team of consulting writers who are asked to interview key players involved in the grant, read the written record, and prepare a report that summarizes what was actually done with the grant funds and what findings, results, and lessons learned emerged. The reports attempt to tell the stories in a manner that lets the reader come to conclusions about what the facts and experiences suggest about success and failure. The grant results reports unit has recently started to prepare topic summaries, also posted on the Foundation's Web site, that synthesize the key outcomes and lessons from reports on a particular topic, such as positive youth development or consumer choice in long-term care.

The grant results reports have emerged as the second most visited area of the Foundation's Web site (just behind the section that describes how to apply for funding). The reports are read by people doing research or planning an initiative that replicates one supported by the Foundation in the past, people interested in knowing what the Foundation funds, and the Foundation's staff members attempting to learn from past lessons to guide current grantmaking.

The Robert Wood Johnson Foundation Anthology, published annually by Jossey-Bass, examines approximately ten topics each year. These topics may be an area of grantmaking, such as health insurance or tobacco policy, or a specific program. Or, in an effort to demystify philanthropy, they may provide an insiders' view of how the Foundation reached decisions or chose one path over another. The writers include award-winning journalists, Foundation staff members, and outside evaluators.

The authors sift through the written record, interview key players, and make site visits. They are asked to write an interesting, jargon-free chapter that lets readers know why the Foundation decided to fund the activity, what the program or programs actually did (or is doing, in the case of existing programs), what has been accomplished, and what lessons can be drawn. The book is distributed to more than ten thousand health care experts, foundation staff members and trustees, and government officials, and is available on the Foundation's Web site.

Taken as a whole, the *Anthology* series, the grant results reports, and publications that emerge from Foundation-funded evaluators (their reports are also available on the Foundation's Web site) offer an extensive record of the Foundation's successes and failures. Serving as a guide to policy makers, health care leaders, researchers, Foundation staff members, and the general public, they represent one way in which the Foundation tries to be accountable to the public and transparent in its grantmaking.

An Assessment

The Foundation prides itself on learning from its programs and its evaluations, constantly attempting to improve how it learns. The evolution of the Foundation's evaluation—from evaluation of individual programs to assessments of the impact of portfolios of grants and the production of an internal scorecard—demonstrates the importance of an institutional culture that promotes continual questioning and desire to learn from past experience.

Even so, the practice of evaluation, assessment, and learning still faces challenges. For example, in its traditional program evaluation, the Foundation needs to be sure that the programs it funds to test new ideas are actually designed so that a convincing test can be conducted. A culture such as that of the Robert Wood Johnson Foundation that wants to choose the best grantees and the best programs—rather than comparing a demonstration site with a control site—can actually work against learning. From a strict learning perspective, sites should be chosen so that a legitimate comparison can be made between places that try an idea and places that do "normal practice."

Another challenge is rationing evaluation dollars so they are spent on cases for which testing and learning are possible. Evaluations are often expensive, and confidentiality requirements and the difficulty of collecting survey data have increased their cost in recent years. When a program is not designed to test a new idea, no evaluation may be needed. The decision *not* to evaluate needs to be made more frequently in order to have money available for more comprehensive evaluations for which testing is possible.

Determining whether a set of Foundation investments have had a causal effect remains a challenge. Currently, performance assessment measures correlation more than causation. Correlation can imply causality when the Foundation's investments are significant enough to be the only likely cause of some event or change. But when the Foundation attempts to affect a complex social situation—such as reducing smoking or improving the quality of health care—it is difficult to know the extent to which the Foundation is responsible for the improvements or whether other factors are the cause.

It is insufficient simply to say that when something positive happens related to a grant program that it is because of the Foundation or its grantees. This expanded sense of impact can be spurious at best. To assess success or failure, the program staff members must be able to articulate the link between the strategy and the expected short-, medium-, and long-term outcomes. Without this type of roadmap, clear assessments will never emerge.

Similarly, the durability of strategy must be considered. On the one hand, it is important for strategy to be flexible enough to react to changes in the environment. On the other hand, if strategies and indicators of success or failure change frequently, then performance assessment is not possible. Constant changes in direction—as opposed to the fine-tuning of a set strategy—generally indicate that a strategy is not working, is not being executed effectively, or was misguided from the start.

Finally, efforts to judge whether the organization itself is working efficiently and effectively require a blend of qualitative assessment and quantitative assessment. The current Robert Wood Johnson Foundation approach perhaps relies too much on quantitative indicators. If the Foundation really wants to know how it is doing, it may need to take the approach of former New York City Mayor Ed Koch and ask in plain language, "How're we doing?" There are many Robert Wood Johnson Foundation-watchers across the country; frank conversations with them could round out the information that the thought leaders' survey provides. Such qualitative information could add an important dimension for the Foundation's board of trustees and senior staff to consider when assessing organizational effectiveness.

The path to developing more effective ways to track and assess performance is the same one the Foundation advises for improving health care quality: continuous quality improvement. Constructing a viable evaluation strategy for a philanthropy is not a one-time building project. It takes constant attention, tinkering, and questioning. While the Robert Wood Johnson Foundation can take pride in its leadership in the field of philanthropic evaluation, it needs to learn from its peers, understand emerging trends in performance assessment, and remain open to evolution in its approaches.

Notes

1. Lavizzo-Mourey, R. "Foreword." To Improve Health and Health Care, Vol. VII: The Robert Wood Johnson Foundation Anthology. San Francisco: Jossey-Bass, 2004.
2. Wielawski, I. "Fighting Back." To Improve Health and Health Care, Vol. VII: The Robert Wood Johnson Foundation Anthology. San Francisco: Jossey-Bass, 2004.
3. Colby, D. C. "Building Research Capacity in the Sciences." To Improve Health and Health Care, Vol. VI: The Robert Wood Johnson Foundation Anthology. San Francisco: Jossey-Bass, 2003.
4. Brown, L. D., and McLaughlin, C. "Constraining Costs at the Community Level: A Critique." Health Affairs, 1990, 9(4), 5–28.
5. Kaplan, R. S., and Norton, D. P. The Balanced Scorecard: Translating Strategy in Action. Cambridge, Mass.: Harvard Business School Press, 1996.

CHAPTER 10

The Sports Philanthropy Project

Digby Diehl

Editors' Introduction

Many corporate foundations choose to make grants to local nonprofit organizations that do charitable work in the community. They often do not consider that by adopting a more strategic approach they could have a sustained and more meaningful impact. Curt Weeden, a former vice president of Johnson & Johnson, has advocated a strategic approach to social investing by corporations that can benefit both the not-for-profit organization and the corporation itself.[1] The foundations (or community relations divisions) of major league sports teams are not generally part of the core business of sports, and they tend to fall into the category of foundations that do not do strategic grantmaking.

In this chapter, Digby Diehl tells the story of the development of the Sports Philanthropy Project. Through this project, the Robert Wood Johnson Foundation worked with foundations established by professional sports teams, helping them develop their philanthropic skills and become more professional in their approach to grantmaking. The project enabled the Foundation to leverage the cachet of professional athletes and teams to further its own health and health care goals. For example, when the Foundation proposed to Major League Soccer that it join in a campaign to enroll uninsured children in the State Children's Health Insurance Program or Medicaid, league officials immediately saw the mutual benefit of such a partnership. Freddie Adu and Jaime Moreno, two stars of the D.C. United team, served as spokespersons for the campaign, and the teams provided children's coverage days at its games, with space for promotion booths, public service announcements, and materials in game books.

Although the Sports Philanthropy Project has encountered some difficulty in establishing an identity of its own, it shows the potential of harnessing the recognition and influence of athletes, teams, and celebrities. For example, salsa musician Willie Colon made a music video concerning children's health insurance, and the cast of NBC's *The Office* made a public service announcement for Cover the Uninsured Week.

Digby Diehl is a best-selling author and frequent contributor to the *Anthology* series. His latest book is *Soapsuds,* written with Finola Hughes.

Notes

1. Weeden, C. *Corporate Social Investing.* San Francisco: Berrett-Koehler, 1998.

—— Standing on the sidelines in Jacksonville's Alltel Stadium at the kickoff of a *Monday Night Football* game between the Jacksonville Jaguars and the Pittsburgh Steelers, the glamour and the excitement are palpable. The ground is literally shaking from twenty-two large men running and smashing into each other in pursuit of a spiraling piece of pigskin that has been kicked high into the air. Cheerleaders leap and perform back flips. Referees in black-and-white striped uniforms blow whistles and wave their arms. Fireworks explode; confetti rains down; and the roar of seventy-three thousand wildly enthusiastic spectators is deafening.

What could this hedonistic, testosterone-driven scene of violence and emotion possibly have to do with the dignified, plush-carpeted, hushed-toned world of a health foundation in Princeton, New Jersey?

"Nothing," answers Joe Marx with a laugh. Marx is the senior Robert Wood Johnson Foundation communications officer and one of the architects of the Sports Philanthropy Project. He continues, "At least, that's what a lot of people at the Foundation thought at first. A typical reaction was, 'These are wealthy owners who build enormous stadiums; the athletes are overpaid. Why should we invest our time and money in *them*?' However, that has changed. Professional sports is big business, yes, but experience has shown that it can also be a big player in driving social change."

The Robert Wood Johnson Foundation has become the first national foundation to try to harness the enormous communications power and public prestige of professional athletics on behalf of health issues. To do so, its staff has had to handle many challenges with patience, diplomacy, and dogged determination over the past nine years. The partnership began with a hodgepodge of well-intentioned ideas, many frustrated efforts, and a few detours. Today, the direction of its work in sports philanthropy has come into clearer focus with specific goals—such as covering the uninsured and fighting childhood obesity—a new administrative structure, and teams committing to sustained health initiatives.

Unlikely Genesis: The Jacksonville Jaguars Scoreboard

The seed of this project was planted in 1995 with a telephone call from Greg Gross, then president of the Jacksonville Jaguars Foundation, to the Robert Wood Johnson Foundation program officer Michael Beachler. Gross had known Beachler from his experiences in the foundation world of Boston, where Gross had worked with several philanthropic groups. He also was aware that the Robert Wood Johnson Foundation had made tobacco control one of its high priorities and had launched some large national programs to combat smoking. Even more specific to sports and tobacco, the Foundation was working with baseball Hall-of-Famer Joe Garagiola on the National Spit Tobacco Education Program.

"As Greg explained to me in our phone conversation, the owners of the Jacksonville Jaguars, Wayne and Delores Weaver, wanted to get rid of the Marlboro scoreboard in the new Jaguars Stadium and replace it with an antitobacco message," Beachler recalls. "The stadium was always a nonsmoking facility, and a large part of the work of the Jaguars Foundation was dedicated to informing children about the dangers of tobacco. The Weavers felt that the scoreboard undermined the work of the Jaguars Foundation."

Gross needed some financial assistance for the Jaguars Foundation to remove and replace the scoreboard. More significantly, however, he recognized the value of having the Robert Wood Johnson imprimatur on the project. Beachler knew that it was a long shot, but it was an innovative proposal. First of all, it was not just a marketing scheme from a sports team. It was part of an ongoing community effort by a sports philanthropy with a proven record, whose work was much larger than this one individual act. The catch was that Gross needed a commitment fast. "After I got off the phone with Greg, I had to make a pitch within the Foundation on one day's notice, with no proposal from the Jaguars to work from," Beachler recalls. "I knew that our president, Steve Schroeder, was a sports fan, and I hoped he would see the potential, so I decided to wing it."

Beachler never got into Schroeder's office. Catching the busy president for a chance meeting in a hallway, he breathlessly pitched the Jaguars idea. "Literally, it was the fastest grant approval I ever got," Beachler says. "He listened, and at the end he said just two words: 'Do it.' Then I raced back to my office and started working with Greg Gross and Joe Marx on the grant proposal."

Schroeder may have said just two words to Beachler, but his thought process about the grant was more complex. "To me, it seemed like a risk worth taking, because it combined two major influences in our culture," Schroeder recalls. "One is sports and the other is the media. The third element I considered is that sports team owners often are beaten up because their athletes do things that are not necessarily emblematic of good citizenship. The Weavers obviously cared about doing some good in their community, and it seemed important to help them. In retrospect, I think it was a substantive grant. If you remove Marlboros as part of the experience of kids going to football games with their dads, you make it a more healthy environment."

On August 1, 1995, the Robert Wood Johnson Foundation board awarded a grant of $137,000 for a new scoreboard and other work with the Jaguars Foundation, as Beachler and Marx were airborne to Jacksonville to help implement the plan. The concept of the Jaguars Don't Smoke campaign came out of their discussions with Gross; Beachler even contributed the image for the sign. "Michael remembered that the Alaska SmokeLess States campaign featured an Iditarod dog stepping on a pack of cigarettes," Marx recalls. "He found the artwork, and they turned it into the image of a jaguar squashing a pack of cigarettes that they used for the sign."

Beyond the Scoreboard: New Health Initiatives in Jacksonville

Shortly after the installation of the new scoreboard, the Jaguars' co-owner, Wayne Weaver, talked with National Football League Commissioner Paul Tagliabue about the NFL contract to publish full-page advertisements for Marlboro cigarettes in the game day programs of all NFL teams. Weaver sought and received permission for the Jaguars to opt out of the Marlboro contract the following year. Two years later, as a result of Weaver's continued discussions with Tagliabue, the NFL cancelled its contract with Philip Morris. This was considered a major step in severing the "glamour" link between smoking and professional sports.

Equally significant for the creation of what was to become the Sports Philanthropy Project, Marx, Beachler, and Gross discussed a range of additional community health ideas sponsored by the Jaguars Foundation. This included their ongoing Honor Rows program, which rewards thousands of Jacksonville children each year with tickets to games, T-shirts, hats, and autograph cards in return for academic distinction or community service and pledges not to use tobacco, alcohol, or drugs.[1] Delores Weaver's Straight Talk program to curb teen pregnancy and AIDS was also marketed through team radio programs and personal appearances.

Back in Princeton, Marx worked with Gross, who was writing another proposal for the Jaguars Foundation. In July 1996, the Robert Wood Johnson Foundation awarded $325,000 to the Jaguars Foundation to expand its youth-oriented tobacco education campaign. Focusing on at-risk children, this grant, with a subsequent renewal, included funds to establish a model elementary school–based health center in Jacksonville, a multiservice youth program in the town's inner city, and programs to increase teaching and accountability regarding tobacco in the schools.

Work Begins with Other Teams: The New Jersey Nets

Beachler, Marx, and Gross soon discussed how the Jaguars' experience could be replicated by other sports teams. "I realized that the Weavers are special people and that the Jaguars Foundation is an exceptional organization, but, most important, I learned how professional sports, as a corporate partner, could be a force for social change like no other," Marx recalls. "Sports teams have such cachet in the community, such market power, and so many other resources. Money is only a part. In the owner's box, I saw political leaders at the state and national level, business leaders in the community—all kinds of decision makers and influential people who were sports fans."

Marx then organized a meeting in 1996 with Foundation staff members and representatives from the New Jersey Nets basketball team, who were interested in hearing how they might participate in the Foundation's programs to reduce tobacco use among young people. As a result of that meeting and subsequent discussions, a $164,000 grant was awarded to the Nets on December 1, 1996, to support a tobacco education campaign called New Jersey Breathes, undertaken in conjunction with the Medical Society of New Jersey.

Coordinated by Gary Sussman, the Nets director of community relations, more than two thousand tickets to Nets games were awarded to children who pledged not to smoke. A mass media campaign, including full-page antismoking ads in every issue of the team program, was mounted. Despite sustained efforts to remove tobacco ads from the Continental Airlines Arena, the Nets' home court, stadium ownership would agree only to move the ads out of camera range for television coverage. Nevertheless, members of the Nets organization estimated that the one-year campaign—the first tobacco-education program ever undertaken by a professional basketball organization—reached an estimated fourteen million people. On December 22, 1997, a follow-up grant of $191,500 was awarded to the Nets for a similar program called Smoking Is an Offensive Foul.

Linking Philanthropies: The First Sports Philanthropy Project Conferences

By 1998, other sports teams had indicated an interest in expanding or starting their own philanthropic work. Gross, the Jaguars Foundation president, suggested that the Robert Wood Johnson Foundation hire Greg Johnson, whom Gross had known from Harvard University, as a consultant to work with other teams. Johnson had worked for seventeen years running the Phillips Brooks House, a human services division of Harvard, and then with Arnold Hiatt, the chief executive officer of the Stride Rite Corporation, on his Stride Rite Charitable Foundation.

In July 1998, Marx and Frank Karel, the Foundation's vice president for communications at the time, invited Johnson to a health communications conference in Princeton. "The three of us talked for a couple of hours afterward, and they pretty much offered me the job then and there," Johnson recalls. "They asked me to survey the field and see what I could find. I started by talking with the Jaguars Foundation, which seemed to be the gold standard for sports philanthropy. Then I talked with the Nets and some of the other sports teams that Joe Marx had already contacted. Within a couple of months, it was obvious that rather than me dealing with them one by one, it would be more efficient to bring the interested teams together so they could talk to one another. We invited representatives from nineteen teams—community relations directors or heads of fledgling foundations—to the Marriott Hotel in Princeton in July 1999.

"We called it our first Sports Philanthropy Project conference, but it was actually more like a think tank—or an AA meeting," Johnson says. "Many of the teams' staff people wanted to gripe that their management simply didn't get philanthropy. We agreed that the discussions would be strictly off the record, and I think that helped us to make real progress understanding the problems that exist in the sports culture."

Johnson was to coordinate efforts to form strategic partnerships between the Robert Wood Johnson Foundation and various team foundations. He was also given the task of helping team foundations to become more "mature," so they would operate more like professional philanthropies with many more years of experience.

"What emerged from that meeting was the need to give interested teams some hands-on technical assistance," Johnson continues. "The Robert Wood Johnson Foundation funded me to work with several teams on some pilot projects to see if I could make a difference. I started with the Nets, and the St. Louis Rams and Baltimore Ravens of the NFL. I lived with each of them for six or seven weeks and built internal infrastructure for communications and networking that they didn't have before." In St. Louis, for example, Johnson worked with the Rams Foundation, which has contributed more than $5 million in cash and in-kind efforts to community work. In 2006, it joined the Healthy Youth Partnership with seventy other organizations to fight childhood obesity through nutrition and physical activity in the St. Louis area schools. The Rams running back Steven Jackson is an active spokesperson for the program. In Baltimore, the Ravens Honor Rows program is based on the Jacksonville program of the same name that Johnson brought to the Ravens' attention; it rewards students for community involvement with tickets to Ravens games. The Ravens have also enlarged their Rookies Youth Football Clinic program, and the Ravens All-Community Team Foundation continues its commitment to high school football and funds numerous field refurbishments.

One of the first meetings Johnson coordinated was between Schroeder and members of the New Jersey Nets corporate staff. At this meeting, Schroeder explained to the Nets new majority owner, Ray Chambers, that to create an effective foundation for his organization he had to hire someone who understood not only the business of sports but also the business of philanthropy. Chambers and his Nets partner, Lewis Katz, embraced this concept. Johnson then worked with Suzanne Spero, executive director of the MCJ Foundation—Chambers' family foundation—to find an appropriately experienced person and to help form a foundation for the Nets. Shortly thereafter, the Nets hired Patricia Goodrich, who had previously worked with the ABC television network in community relations.

Although it was clear at this early point that the Foundation was correct in its initial recognition of the potential in sports philanthropy, it was also clear that it would take time to fulfill that potential. In 2000, the Sports Philanthropy Project consisted only of Greg Johnson, his temporary assistant, and a summer intern. That summer, the name "Sports Philanthropy Project" was used for the first time at a Sports Philanthropy Project conference held in Boston. Attended by representatives of twenty-two franchises in baseball, basketball, football, and hockey, it featured the noted Harvard professor and child psychiatrist Robert Coles as the keynote speaker.

Teamwork

Building on the momentum of the 1999 and 2000 conferences, Johnson began expanding the project. Discussions at the first conference made clear the need for education about philanthropy at every level of sports teams, from ownership to community relations organizers. The second conference emphasized the need for technical assistance in helping teams to set up a philanthropic framework. The Sports Philanthropy Project Web site was launched shortly thereafter. Johnson also hired Van Le, an attorney from the Boston law firm of Ropes & Gray. Le came to the Sports Philanthropy Project from a diverse background that included work in the public defender's office, in a refugee camp in the Philippines, and with Johnson at the Phillips Brooks House.

"Candidly, in the early days, sports teams were reluctant to allow philanthropy consultants in the door," Le says. "They were afraid of criticism, so we added client confidentiality agreements to our relationships, which made the teams more comfortable."

The Golden State Warriors

Le's first project, in 2001, was as a consultant to the NBA's Golden State Warriors, headquartered in Oakland, California. The team had created the Golden State Warriors Foundation in 1997; since then, with CEO Christopher Cohan's wife, Angela, as president of the Foundation, they have distributed more than $1.5 million to nonprofit organizations. "When I worked with them, the Warriors had already established an afterschool program for children in Oakland, as well as a junior basketball league—with thousands of kids playing under their sponsorship," Le recalls. "They also contributed to anti–substance abuse initiatives and promoted literacy. In our work, we try to help teams look at the impact of what they are doing. We help them to clarify their mission and to focus on organizing principles. One result of these discussions with the Warriors was that they worked more closely with the Alameda County Public Health program to promote physical activity." In conjunction with Kaiser Permanente, the Warriors developed a Get Fit program to fight childhood obesity. Team members visit elementary, middle, and high schools to promote healthy eating and active lifestyles.

Reds, Burn, Bills

Le next spent several months advising three more teams: Major League Baseball's Cincinnati Reds, the Dallas Burn of Major League Soccer, and the National Football League's Buffalo Bills. "In Cincinnati, we were able to help the Reds take a more active role in community relations, to set up an effective team foundation, and to begin a youth program called the Reds Rookie Success League," Le notes. The Reds Rookie Success League targets at-risk eight- to eleven-year-olds, offering a summer of coed baseball that is frequently visited by Reds players. It also includes medical, dental, and vision screening.

The Dallas Burn soccer team (later renamed FC Dallas) developed programming within the Latino community that supports youth soccer and aggressive anti–substance abuse efforts. Currently, the FC Dallas Foundation, through its Kicks for Kids program, distributes one thousand game tickets to community groups and schools to reward inner-city, at-risk, and disadvantaged children in the Dallas-Fort Worth area who have given community service or made pledges to abstain from tobacco, drugs, and alcohol use.

The Buffalo Bills became the first team in the NFL to build a facility dedicated to youth football on the same grounds as the team headquarters. The team supports an active program of youth football and offers tickets to Bills games as a reward for community service efforts through the Buffalo Bills Youth Foundation.

Leveraging Pro Sports for Health

As the Sports Philanthropy Project developed, its activities became more closely aligned with those of the Robert Wood Johnson Foundation, and it was able to bring the star power of professional sports to important health issues such as combating childhood obesity and expanding health insurance coverage for children.

Lisa Willis, the director of development, began in mid-2001 as the Sports Philanthropy Project director of marketing and communications; like all of the members of the small Sports Philanthropy Project team, she was immediately wearing many hats. "As the title suggests, I began by working on marketing brochures and expanding the Web site," she said. "The second part of my job was organizing our conferences." Willis is especially proud of the Sports Philanthropy Project's work with two Foundation-funded social marketing campaigns: Cover the Uninsured Week and the Covering Kids & Families communications campaign. Her work with Major League Soccer to promote health insurance for children illustrates the way in which professional sports and philanthropy can collaborate for the public good. Willis worked closely with the Robert Wood Johnson Foundation's coverage team and with the GMMB public relations agency (a subsidiary of Fleishman-Hillard), to enlist support from Major League Soccer and, initially, its teams in New York, Los Angeles, San Jose, and Chicago.

It was a win-win situation. Major League Soccer, striving to develop a market in the United States, gained credibility from its Foundation-connected work to improve community health. For its part, the Robert Wood Johnson Foundation was able to leverage the reach of Major League Soccer in the Latino community, which has a disproportionately high number of uninsured children. All twelve professional soccer teams, as well as Major League Soccer itself, now engage in promotional efforts to support Covering Kids & Families. These efforts include

- Events at schools with soccer players
- Public service announcements during games
- Informational materials about health insurance at stadium booths
- Ad space in Major League Soccer game programs

Alisha Greenberg, manager of client services, joined the Sports Philanthropy Project in January 2002 and began to work with Willis on the Web site, conferences, and, later, social marketing campaigns. The July 2002 Sports Philanthropy Project Conference attracted more than 120 professional sports team and athlete foundation representatives to Chicago, where Greenberg first met representatives from the Chicago Fire soccer team. She later had the honor of kicking out the first ball as part of the Fire's Children's Health Care Coverage Day, which she had helped to organize. The Chicago Fire team foundation has developed a pilot program, the Active Kids Initiative, a comprehensive school- and community-based effort to fight childhood obesity—a high priority of the Robert Wood Johnson Foundation—in three of the most at-risk Chicago communities: South Shore, South Lawndale, and Bridgeview.

2003–2006: Challenges and Focus

By 2003, the Sports Philanthropy Project had received Robert Wood Johnson Foundation funding for five years. The Foundation traditionally uses its resources as start-up financing for programs, with the expectation that recipients will eventually become self-sustaining. Within the Foundation, there was discussion about whether the Sports Philanthropy Project really had the potential to harness professional sports to promote better health, whether it would be able to become self-sufficient, whether it was organized properly, and whether further investment would yield the health results that the Foundation was seeking. "These discussions led us to suggest that the Sports Philanthropy Project bring in outside experts to evaluate its progress to date and help it assess where it was going; that it develop a long-range plan; and that it become self-sustaining—and in doing so, that it consider various scenarios about the future, both with and without financial support from the Robert Wood Johnson Foundation," Joe Marx says. The evaluation and strategic planning was contracted to Development Resources, Inc., or DRI, and was headed by Jennifer Dunlap, former senior vice president of development for the American Red Cross.

Even as it was telling the Sports Philanthropy Project that the time had come to consider all of its options for the future, the Foundation awarded the Project roughly two million dollars in 2003 and 2004 to continue the work it had been doing, and to carry out the evaluation and strategic planning process. Under the terms of the grant awards, the goals of the Project were refined to address two health concerns—coverage of the uninsured and childhood obesity—and links with additional teams were to be forged. The grant specified that the Sports Philanthropy Project was to continue its collaboration with the Covering Kids & Families communications campaign and develop programs to promote physical activity and reduce childhood obesity in Phoenix and two additional cities.

Potential Support from the W.K. Kellogg Foundation

As a result of the Robert Wood Johnson Foundation's instruction to seek ways of becoming self-sustaining and the uncertainty about the Project's long-term financial future, in late 2003 the Sports Philanthropy Project submitted a solicited proposal to the W.K. Kellogg Foundation "to strengthen and promote philanthropy among athletes as a strategy for community engagement and leadership development among young people." The application was successful, and in February 2004 the Kellogg

Foundation awarded the Sports Philanthropy Project a four-year grant for $3.5 million. The grant had one major proviso: Kellogg was to take over the running of the Sports Philanthropy Project.

The Sports Philanthropy Project was at a crossroads. As Greg Johnson explains it, there was a financial crisis looming because the future of Robert Wood Johnson sponsorship was uncertain. "I had to look at my staff and the future of the organization," Johnson says. "If support from that foundation was coming to an end, turning the Sports Philanthropy Project over to another funder would be the responsible thing to do.

"The problem was that Kellogg wanted us to work exclusively with individual athlete foundations, and Robert Wood Johnson wanted us to continue the work we had been doing primarily with teams and organizations representing groups of teams," Johnson continues. "Simultaneously, we had been moving toward setting ourselves up as a separate nonprofit corporation and forming a board. One of the first questions we put to the board was whether these two grants could be symbiotic or whether we had to choose. The board, in conjunction with an outside consultant, decided that we should continue to work with teams, as we had been, and to continue our relationship with the Robert Wood Johnson Foundation." For its part, the Kellogg Foundation went forward with its intention to work with individual sports figures and their personal foundations. It reorganized its grant as the Athlete Legacy League and continued independently. In 2006, the Robert Wood Johnson Foundation awarded $3.5 million to the Sports Philanthropy Project to continue its work through 2010.

Understandably, no one wanted to go on record regarding a widely known problem of individual athlete foundations: they can be capricious and unreliable. There are certainly impressive examples of athlete philanthropy, including the New York Giants football star Tiki Barber, the golfer Tiger Woods, the cyclist Lance Armstrong, the tennis icon Andre Agassi, and the Yankees' star Derek Jeter. They appear, however, to be commendable exceptions. "Even among those athletes with charitable leanings, the record is uneven," Lynn Zinser pointed out in a thoughtful *New York Times* article on the topic.[2] "Many never advance beyond making appearances, contributing nothing more than time and autographs. Some spend their energy and resources on events like star-studded charity golf tournaments." Others, such as Michael Jordan, begin with good intentions and discover that the foundation is being mishandled or that little money reaches the intended recipients. Jordan closed his foundation in 1996.

Sports Philanthropy Project's Giant Step Forward in Arizona

Early in 2003, Steve Patterson got in touch with the Sports Philanthropy Project on behalf of the Arizona Sports and Tourism Authority, or AZSTA. Patterson, a UCLA basketball star under coach John Wooden and former professional player with the Cleveland Cavaliers and the Chicago Bulls, was working as a consultant to AZSTA through his company, Patterson Sports Ventures. He found Greg Johnson at the Sports Philanthropy Project through the Internet, and after several conversations he invited Johnson to give the welcoming address at AZSTA's First Annual Youth and Amateur Sports Summit.

AZSTA had been created in 2000 to handle four very large interrelated projects:

- Construction of a new $380 million stadium for the Arizona Cardinals
- Administration of the Cactus League spring training facilities for Major League Baseball, including refurbishment of existing stadiums and building of more stadiums and facilities
- Funding of tourism development in Maricopa County
- Distribution of a projected $73.5 million over thirty years for youth sports facilities

These projects had been approved under the terms of Proposition 302, a controversial bond issue that was passed by a narrow majority of Arizona voters.

"The group I addressed was a cross-section of the public, many of whom were unhappy with the Cardinals stadium and AZSTA," Johnson recalls. "I was candid. I asked those people to make demands of the team, of AZSTA, and to use this opportunity in a wise fashion rather than squander it. I also offered to have the Sports Philanthropy Project do some *pro bono* work with Steve to design ways to make this situation work for the entire community."

The offices of Ted Ferris, the CEO of AZSTA, are in the colossal new Cardinals stadium. This state-of-the-art facility has features that wow all first-time visitors. Most astonishing, its natural grass playing field is fully retractable; beneath it lies 160,000 square feet of column-free space, ideal for conventions and trade shows. The entire roof rolls back for open-air events; otherwise, the high-tech environment is fully air-conditioned against the blazing Arizona sun. With 63,500 fixed seats and 10,000 more that can be added, this stadium is ready for the annual Fiesta Bowl, the Super Bowl (in 2008), and almost any gathering or event you can name.

"I think we are making this situation work rather well for the entire community," Ferris comments. "We have the world's biggest and best multipurpose arena, and it is already bringing in tourism tax dollars for Arizona. We are continuing and enlarging the spring training facilities for Major League Baseball teams, with two proposals for building new stadiums, as well as rehabilitating the existing stadiums. I can't take credit for putting together the excellent community efforts—that credit goes to Steve Patterson, Greg Johnson, and Van Le—but I will take some credit for listening and being open to their good ideas.

In working with the community, there was a great deal of initial resistance to be overcome. "I was asked to go to Phoenix to help put together a coalition of people who would be interested in working on childhood obesity," Van Le says. When he arrived, he found that the term *coalition* was premature and that a lot of people were not satisfied with the AZSTA's $73 million grant program."

This was new territory for the Sports Philanthropy Project. AZSTA clearly was not a team foundation. However, the problems of understanding focus and sustained effort on behalf of a community issue were the same. Le realized that AZSTA was not really set up to handle this undertaking. He suggested the formation of an independent, broad-based community coalition tasked with more than just handing out money.

"The mission I proposed was sponsoring physical activity and fighting childhood obesity in Phoenix," Le recalls. "We suggested that the coalition be composed of professionals in the field, from public health to youth organizations to park districts. David Morse, the Robert Wood Johnson Foundation's vice president for communications, arranged a one-time grant of $75,000 to get the coalition going, which was matched by the Arizona Cardinals and AZSTA. At that point, we created the Maricopa Council on Youth Sports and Physical Activity—MCYSPA, which is pronounced 'Mickey Spa'—and hired Shawna Bradlich as the executive director. AZSTA administers the grants, but the rest is handled by MCYSPA. The Robert Wood Johnson Foundation's participation gave the project credibility with other foundations."

Bradlich notes, "By vouching for the validity of such an innovative concept—a community body participating in the allocation of tax dollars—the Foundation triggered a domino effect for other funders at the table."

MCYSPA ostensibly functions as an advisory group to AZSTA. As a result, although 100 percent of its recommendations are accepted by the AZSTA board, MCYSPA is not set up as a separate 501(c)(3) nonprofit organization. Consequently, executive director Shawna Bradlich works with the Arizona Community Foundation, which encompasses more than eight hundred funds with combined assets of $560 million, according to Deborah Whitehurst, chief operating officer of the community foundation. "We are the fiscal agent for MCYSPA, but we also are sometimes involved in programmatic advisory roles," Whitehurst says. "We are able to reach out to other people who might want to fund the coalition or partner in certain projects."

An example of coalition funding is presented by Dr. Jonathan Weisbuch, former public health director of Maricopa County: "When I joined the board of MCYSPA, it became clear that by joining forces with this organization, not only would we have an opportunity for funding, but we would also have an opportunity for input. For example, one of the exciting things that Steve Patterson had already organized for MCYSPA funding was an extraordinary Geographic Information System program at Arizona State University. One of the computer guys there showed us how he could identify on the map of Maricopa County all of the athletic fields and exercise resources available to individuals, and he could link them to information such as field schedules, when the games were played, the names of coaches, and so forth. You can cross-reference that with the population density, the ethnic mix of people in the area, and all sorts of information with health implications. There are more than two thousand facilities and programs already mapped. They are working on a program like that for the whole state of Arizona."

Everywhere in Maricopa County, there are projects funded by AZSTA. At the Golden Gate Community Center, AZSTA has funded the renovation of a large gymnasium, which is shared by children and adults—all into exercise. "At Avondale Friendship Park," says Don Davis, the director of Avondale's Parks, Recreation, and Libraries Department, "we established these multipurpose fields three years ago, and now they are in use so often year-round that we have to reserve time to allow the grass to grow back. In 2006, AZSTA provided the funding to set up night

---

Steve Patterson began his basketball career at UCLA as a key player on three national championship teams. After graduation, Patterson played for the Cleveland Cavaliers and the Chicago Bulls and coached several basketball teams in Arizona, including Arizona State University's. He formed Patterson Sports Ventures with his wife, Carlette, to link players, teams, and sports foundations with social causes. Shortly after his death from lung cancer on July 28, 2004, at the age of fifty-six, the Robert Wood Johnson Foundation and the Sports Philanthropy Project established an award in his name.[3] Patterson's coach, the legendary John Wooden, observes, "It is quite appropriate that an award of this type, one that represents someone committed to giving, be named for Steve Patterson, who truly spent his life giving."

"Steve saw his philanthropy work as an extension of coaching basketball," Carlette Patterson says. "It is *life* coaching. If you think about the amount of money that the athletes and the leagues have available today, it is enough to make incredible changes in our society. When athletes come from the areas that need change, you are asking them to get involved and give back to their communities, their cousins, their neighbors, their friends, kids just like them.

"Sports philanthropy is basically in its rookie years," she observes. "It is first-generation money. This is a huge paradigm shift—even talking 'sports philanthropy' is a new language that we didn't have ten years ago. That is what's so exciting about this field, especially now that the Robert Wood Johnson Founda-

lights on several fields, so that we have more hours available to the community." Similar multiuse fields surround the Cardinals stadium in the suburb of Glendale, which are maintained jointly by the City of Glendale, the Fiesta Bowl parking authority, and AZSTA. At the South Mountain YMCA, located in an area identified as having a high prevalence of childhood obesity, the Arizona Cardinals' All Kids Can Club is providing healthy exercise classes and nutrition counseling to children aged five to thirteen.

At the Peoria Sports Complex, a spring training facility for the Seattle Mariners and the San Diego Padres, Jon Richardson, the executive director of the Peoria Diamond Club and a MCYSPA board member, explains how his organization works with the coalition: "We're a nonprofit that operates the ballpark and the training facilities. During the spring

tion and the Sports Philanthropy Project are engaged. We are just beginning to see the best part of sports helping the whole society. I am really proud that this award continues Steve's legacy."

The first Steve Patterson Sports Philanthropy Award was presented in 2005 to the Philadelphia Eagles Youth Partnership for its pioneering Eagles Eye Mobile program, which provides free eye exams, glasses, and other services to young people who otherwise could not afford them. The program was begun at the initiative of Jermane Mayberry, an Eagles guard and tackle from 1996 to 2004, who donated $118,000 to launch the program. Mayberry suffers from amblyopia, or underdeveloped optic nerve, and is legally blind in his left eye. He wanted other children to have early eye exams, which might have prevented his condition. Since 1996, the Eye Mobile has examined more than one hundred thousand children and continues operating today.

John Lumpkin, a Robert Wood Johnson Foundation senior vice president, called the Jacksonville Jaguars Foundation "a model philanthropy" at pregame ceremonies for the 2006 Steve Patterson Sports Philanthropy Award in Jacksonville, Florida. The award received national attention on the ESPN *Cold Pizza* show following a *Monday Night Football* game. Citing the Jaguars Don't Smoke program, Lumpkin noted, "You have applied the power of your position in the community strategically and effectively—facing tough issues, seeking solutions over the long haul, and improving the health and strength of the Jacksonville community."

training season, the two teams play about thirty home games in a row between them. We'll see about 115,000 people in those thirty days, and our biggest crowds can be up to 13,000. In the off-season, we have concerts, youth games, local and out-of-area tournaments and championship games, graduations, RV shows, boat shows, custom car shows, and a big Fourth of July fireworks show. We generate a lot of tourism dollars, and we also do a lot for the community. The money we make we give to youth organizations in Arizona."

According to Richardson, the facility gives away 100 percent of its profits to youth organizations, some of it through MCYSPA. "Jon is a major player in another initiative of MCYSPA," Shawna Bradlich notes. "The Summer Youth Program Fund is a new coalition, made up of eleven funders, including the Peoria Diamond Club, that will award about half a million dollars in 2007 for summer youth programs, and we are just getting started. He has brought in his Fiesta Bowl contacts, his Phoenix International Raceway contacts, and his friends at the other spring training facilities. This allows us to offer more programming support, whereas our role with AZSTA is more facility support."

2006 and Beyond: The Future of the Sports Philanthropy Project

We live in a celebrity-driven culture, and it is natural for many people to be dazzled by the accomplishments of individual athletes. Teams and athletes have important roles to play as model citizens and community leaders. They can have tremendous impact, perhaps more than politicians. To channel this respect—adoration, even—into something that will benefit the health of the community, the Sports Philanthropy Project has worked with teams and with community coalitions associated with teams. The idea is a winning one, but the execution has not lived up to the full promise until recently.

Since its inception, the Sports Philanthropy Project has carried out a variety of well-intentioned activities, some of which had an impact, others of which did not. The project did not have a consistent focus and lacked an identity. The evaluation by DRI, which was presented in April 2005, zeroed in on this problem. "What is the Sports Philanthropy

Project—A consulting practice? An association? A membership organization? A technical resource?" asked team representatives and other stakeholders quoted in the report. The report concluded that "the Sports Philanthropy Project must define and commit to who it is and what it will do."

After the 2005 DRI evaluation, the Sports Philanthropy Project ratcheted up its efforts to develop a clear identity. Greg Johnson articulated what he saw as the role of the Sports Philanthropy Project. "I began to understand that sports philanthropy is really corporate philanthropy with a special twist," he says. "Sports teams are large corporate franchises that also have special assets that allow them to have considerable impact on the culture. I learned to see our role as middlemen who partner with the teams to leverage their special assets on behalf of public health missions created by the Robert Wood Johnson Foundation. For example, initially we worked on substance abuse and the uninsured, but as the Foundation added a focus on physical activity and obesity issues for youth, so did we."

The Project has been working to develop a coherent strategy and structure that will raise the ethical standards of teams, serve the community by improving health, and provide the Project with a clear and understandable identity that will give it the visibility and credibility to attract funds. The Sports Philanthropy Project's work in Phoenix is serving as something of a model for teams and community coalitions. As Joe Marx points out, "In many ways, the Phoenix project is a key to the future of the Sports Philanthropy Project. It is important because in Phoenix, sports teams joined hands with local businesses, government, foundations, and other community groups to focus on the problem of childhood obesity. It is important because the commitments are long-range and already are beginning to show benefits for the health of children." For its part, the Robert Wood Johnson Foundation's $3.5 million grant, awarded in 2006, will ensure the Project's financial stability through 2010 and will enable it to help the professional sports teams' foundations become more strategic and effective in their activities.

The Sports Philanthropy Project has formed a board and become a 501(c)(3) nonprofit organization. "There have been discussions about renaming the organization once we cease to be a 'project' of the Robert Wood Johnson Foundation, and I think that will happen," Johnson says. To channel the power of professional sports in the service of social change, the Sports Philanthropy Project is focusing on a number of discrete activities:

- Coalition building and program development
- Social marketing
- Direct technical assistance
- The Steve Patterson Sports Philanthropy Award
- Conferences, workshops, and "webinars"
- A Web site

Recently, several encouraging developments have occurred at the Sports Philanthropy Project:

- Greg Johnson was invited to participate in a symposium on "Corporate Social Responsibility in Professional Sport" at the 2007 North American Society for Sport Management conference.
- The 2007 Steve Patterson Sports Philanthropy Award was presented at the Associated Press Sports Editors convention in St. Louis to both the Memphis Grizzlies Charitable Foundation and the Moyer Foundation.
- A nationwide survey of sports philanthropy conducted by the Sports Philanthropy Project was published in 2007.

The most recent news, according to Greg Johnson, is that "we have met with executives of Major League Baseball and submitted a proposal to examine the philanthropic efforts of all the teams and work with the owners in thirty cities. That could be a huge step forward in sports philanthropy—if it happens."

As it has been from the start, the potential of the Sports Philanthropy Project is great. Perhaps the best example is that of its collaboration with Major League Soccer, which has a unique ability to reach an audience of uninsured Latino children that is particularly important to the Robert Wood Johnson Foundation. Although only some of that potential has been reached to date, more can be expected in the future. The optimistic vision of the Sports Philanthropy Project is that sports teams in the United

States can become engines of healthy physical activity, sportsmanship, and good citizenship. It is a vision worth pursuing.

Notes

1. Parker, S. "The Sports Philanthropy Project: A Training Ground for Sports Foundations." *ADVANCES, The Robert Wood Johnson Foundation Quarterly Newsletter,* 2002, *2.*
2. Zinser, L. "Athletes Practice the Giveback." *New York Times,* Nov. 13, 2006. Another recent article offers individual athlete foundation financial information: Bondy, F. "Charity Cases: Athlete's Gifts Don't Always Build Strong Foundations." *The Olympian,* Feb. 26, 2007.
3. More information about the Steve Patterson Sports Philanthropy Award is available at the web site www.stevepattersonaward.org/.

The Editors

Stephen L. Isaacs, J.D., is a partner in Isaacs/Jellinek, a San Francisco-based consulting firm, and president of Health Policy Associates, Inc. A former professor of public health at Columbia University and founding director of its Development Law and Policy Program, he has written extensively for professional and popular audiences. His book, *The Consumer's Legal Guide to Today's Health Care*, was reviewed as "the single best guide to the health care system in print today." His articles have been widely syndicated and have appeared in law reviews and health policy journals. He also provides technical assistance internationally on health law, civil society, and social policy. A graduate of Brown University and Columbia Law School, Isaacs served as vice president of International Planned Parenthood's Western Hemisphere Region, practiced health law, and spent four years in Thailand as a program officer for the U.S. Agency for International Development.

David C. Colby, Ph.D., is the vice president of research and evaluation at the Robert Wood Johnson Foundation. Previously, he was the deputy director of research and evaluation, the deputy director of the health care group, interim team leader for the quality team, and team leader for the coverage team at the Foundation. He came to the Foundation in January 1998 after nine years of service with the Medicare Payment Advisory Commission and the Physician Payment Review Commission, where he was deputy director. Earlier he taught at the University of Maryland Baltimore County, Williams College, and State University College at Buffalo. Colby's published research has focused on Medicaid and Medicare, media coverage of AIDS, and various topics in political science. He was an associate editor of the *Journal of Health Politics, Policy and Law* from 1995 to 2002. He received his doctorate in political science from the University of Illinois, master of arts from Ohio University, and a bachelor of arts from Ohio Wesleyan University.

The Contributors

Paul Brodeur was a staff writer at the *New Yorker* for many years. During that time, he alerted the nation to the public health hazard posed by asbestos, to depletion of the ozone layer by chlorofluorocarbons, and to the harmful effects of microwave radiation and power-frequency electromagnetic fields. His work has been acknowledged with a National Magazine Award and the Journalism Award of the American Association for the Advancement of Science. The United Nations Environment Program has named him to its Global 500 Roll of Honor for outstanding environmental achievements.

Will Bunch is the senior writer for the *Philadelphia Daily News* and its former political writer, gaining national recognition for his scoops on the 9/11 attacks and the war in Iraq. Before coming to Philadelphia, Bunch was a key member of the *New York Newsday* team that won the 1992 Pulitzer Prize for spot news reporting. His magazine articles have appeared in a number of national and regional publications, including the *New York Times Magazine,* and he is a contributing editor at his alma mater's *Brown Alumni Magazine.* Bunch is also the author of the critically praised 1994 book *Jukebox America: Down Back Streets and Blue Highways in Search of the Country's Greatest Jukebox.*

Digby Diehl is a writer, literary collaborator, and television, print, and internet journalist. His book credits include the recent novel *Soapsuds,* written with Finola Hughes; *Angel on My Shoulder,* the autobiography of singer Natalie Cole; *The Million Dollar Mermaid,* the autobiography of MGM star Esther Williams; *Tales from the Crypt,* the history of the popular comic book, movie, and television series; and *A Spy for All Seasons,* the autobiography of former CIA officer Duane Clarridge. For eleven years, Diehl was the literary correspondent for ABC-TV's *Good Morning America*, and he was recently the book editor for the *Home Page* show on MSNBC. Previously the entertainment editor for KCBS television in Los Angeles, he was a writer for the Emmys and for the soap opera *Santa Barbara*, book editor of the *Los Angeles Herald Examiner,* editor-in-chief of art book publisher Harry N. Abrams, and the founding book editor of the *Los Angeles Times Book Review*. Diehl holds a master of arts in theatre from UCLA and a bachelor of arts in American studies from Rutgers University, where he was a Henry Rutgers Scholar.

Kelly A. Hunt is a senior program director at the New York State Health Foundation with over fourteen years of experience in developing, managing, and funding health care policy analysis and working at the community level. Most recently, Hunt served as a research and evaluation officer at the Robert Wood Johnson Foundation, where she led the team responsible for the organization's scorecard, an annual assessment of the Foundation's impact. She is a coauthor of numerous health services research articles that have appeared in journals such as *Health Affairs, Health Services Research*, the *Milbank Quarterly*, and the *Annals of Emergency Medicine*. She holds a master of public policy from Georgetown University and a bachelor of arts from Villanova University.

Paul S. Jellinek, Ph.D., is a partner in Isaacs-Jellinek, a San Francisco-based consulting firm that works with private foundations and other nonprofit organizations committed to the public good, and is a senior fellow of Health Policy Associates, Inc. A former vice president of the Robert Wood Johnson Foundation, where he served for almost twenty years, he was actively involved in the development and management of some of its major national initiatives in the areas of child and adolescent health, substance abuse, AIDS, and volunteerism, and chaired its working groups in the areas of health care access and community health. A graduate of the University of Pennsylvania, the University of South Florida, and the University of North Carolina School of Public Health, Jellinek was trained in health administration and health care economics, and his articles have appeared in a variety of health and policy journals.

James R. Knickman, Ph.D., is president and chief executive officer of the New York State Health Foundation, which focuses on improving access to health care and public health and expansion of insurance coverage for New Yorkers. For fourteen years Knickman was vice president for research and evaluation at the Robert Wood Johnson Foundation, where he oversaw a range of grants and national programs supporting research and policy analysis to better understand forces that can improve health status and delivery of health care. In addition, he was in charge of developing formal evaluations of national programs supported by the Foundation and the Foundation's performance assessment system. During the 1999–2000 academic year he held a Regents' Lectureship at the University of California, Berkeley. Previously, Knickman was on the faculty of the Robert Wagner Graduate School of Public Service at New York University. At NYU he was the founding director of a university-wide research center focused on urban health care. His publications include research on a range of health care topics, with particular emphasis on issues related to financing and delivering long-term care. He has served on numerous health-related advisory committees at the state and local levels and spent a year working at New York City's Office of Management and Budget. Currently, he chairs the board of trustees of the Robert Wood Johnson University Health System in New Brunswick. He completed his undergraduate work at Fordham University and received his doctorate in public policy analysis from the University of Pennsylvania.

Risa Lavizzo-Mourey, M.D., M.B.A., is the fourth president and chief executive officer of the Robert Wood Johnson Foundation, a position she assumed in January 2003. Under her leadership, the Foundation implemented a defining framework that focuses its mission to improve the health and health care of all Americans and set bold objectives in nursing, health care disparities, and childhood obesity as well as improving public health and quality in the health care system. She originally joined the staff in April 2001 as the senior vice president and director of the health care group. Prior to coming to the Foundation, Lavizzo-Mourey was the Sylvan Eisman Professor of Medicine and Health Care Systems at the University of Pennsylvania, as well as director of the Institute on Aging. Lavizzo-Mourey was the deputy administrator of the Agency for

Health Care Policy and Research, now known as the Agency for Health Care Research and Quality. Lavizzo-Mourey is the author of numerous articles and several books, and the recipient of many awards and honorary doctorates. She frequently appears on national radio and television. A member of the Institute of Medicine of the National Academy of Sciences, she earned her medical degree at Harvard Medical School followed by a master's in business administration at the University of Pennsylvania's Wharton School. After completing a residency in internal medicine at Brigham and Women's Hospital in Boston, Massachusetts, Lavizzo-Mourey was a Robert Wood Johnson Clinical Scholar at the University of Pennsylvania, where she also received her geriatrics training.

Susan McGrath has been a writer of creative nonfiction for twenty-three years, specializing in natural history, the environment, and human-health-related environmental subjects. She wrote a news-you-can-use environmental column called "The Household Environmentalist" that ran in the *Seattle Times* for eight years and was syndicated nationally by the Los Angeles Times Syndicate. Her work appears in *Audubon, National Geographic, Smithsonian,* and other magazines.

Fen Montaigne is a journalist and author whose work has appeared frequently in *National Geographic* magazine. He also has written for *Smithsonian, Outside, Forbes,* and *Audubon* magazines, as well as for the *Wall Street Journal.* Before becoming a freelance writer in 1996, Montaigne worked for the *Philadelphia Inquirer* for fifteen years, where he served as the paper's Moscow correspondent from 1990 to 1993, covering the collapse of the Soviet Union. Now specializing in environmental and science writing, Montaigne has authored or coauthored four books, including the travel-adventure book *Reeling in Russia* and *Medicine by Design,* which tells the story of biomedical engineering. Montaigne is currently at work on a book about the rapid warming of the Antarctic Peninsula and its effect on Adelie penguins and other wildlife. He is a recipient of a 2006 Guggenheim Foundation fellowship to support his research and writing of the book on Antarctica. Montaigne has been a finalist for the Pulitzer Prize in feature writing and has won several Overseas Press Club awards for his reporting from around the globe.

Carolyn Newbergh is a Northern California writer who has covered health care trends and policy issues for more than twenty years. Her freelance work has appeared in numerous print and online publications. As a reporter for the *Oakland Tribune,* she wrote articles on health care delivery for the poor, as well as emergency room violence, AIDS, and the impact of crack cocaine on the children of addicts. She was also an investigative reporter for the *Tribune,* winning prestigious honors for a series on how consultants intentionally cover up earthquake hazards in California.

Irene M. Wielawski is a health care journalist with twenty years' experience as a staff writer for daily newspapers, including the *Providence Journal-Bulletin* and the *Los Angeles Times,* where she was a member of the investigations team. She has written extensively on problems of access to care among the poor and uninsured and on other socioeconomic issues in American medicine. From 1994 through 2000, Wielawski—with a research grant from the Robert Wood Johnson Foundation—tracked the experiences of the medically uninsured in twenty-five states following the demise of President Clinton's health reform plan. Other projects in health care journalism since then include helping to develop a pediatric medicine program for public television as well as freelance writing and editing for various publications, including the *New York Times*, the *Los Angeles Times*, and science and policy journals. Wielawski has been a finalist for the Pulitzer Prize for medical reporting, among other solo honors. She is a founder of the Association of Health Care Journalists and a graduate of Vassar College.

Index

D

Table of Contents

To Improve Health and Health Care 1997

Table of Contents

To Improve Health and Health Care 1998–1999

Table of Contents

To Improve Health and Health Care 2000

—≋— Table of Contents

To Improve Health and Health Care 2001

Table of Contents

To Improve Health and Health Care Volume V

Table of Contents

To Improve Health and Health Care Volume VI

Table of Contents

To Improve Health and Health Care Volume VII

Table of Contents

To Improve Health and Health Care Volume VIII

Table of Contents

To Improve Health and Health Care Volume IX

Table of Contents

To Improve Health and Health Care Volume X